ECG diagnosis

Self Assessment
Volume II

Edward K. Chung, M.D., F.A.C.P., F.A.C.C.

Professor of Medicine
Jefferson Medical College of
Thomas Jefferson University
and
Director of the Heart Station
Thomas Jefferson University Hospital
Philadelphia, Pennsylvania

ECG diagnosis

Self Assessment
Volume II

Medical Department
HARPER & ROW, PUBLISHERS • Hagerstown, Maryland
New York, San Francisco, London

DRUG DOSAGE

The author and publisher have exerted every effort to ensure that drug selection and dosage set forth in this text are in accord with current recommendations and practice at the time of publication. However, in view of ongoing research, changes in government regulations, and the constant flow of information relating to drug therapy and drug reactions, the reader is urged to check the package insert for each drug for any change in indications and dosage and for added warnings and precautions. This is particularly important when the recommended agent is a new and/or infrequently employed drug.

77 78 79 80 81 82   10 9 8 7 6 5 4 3 2 1

Library of Congress Cataloging in Publication Data (Revised)
Chung, Edward K
    ECG diagnosis.

    Vol. 2 by E. K. Chung.
    Includes bibliographies.
    1. Electrocardiography—Cases, clinical reports, statistics. I. Chung, Donald K., joint author. II. Title. [DNLM: 1. Electrocardiography. WG140 C559e 1972]
RC683.5.E5C46   616.1′2′0754   75–185644
ISBN 0–06–140638–4 (v. 1)

To my wife, Lisa
and
my children, Linda and Christopher

Contents

Preface

		Case Nos.
1	Normal Variants	1–9
2	Chamber Enlargement (Hypertrophy)	10–27
3	Myocardial Ischemia, Injury, and Infarction	28–53
4	Myocarditis and Pericarditis	54–70
5	Disturbances of Sinus Impulse Formation and Conduction	71–82
6	Atrial Arrhythmias	83–111
7	Atrioventricular (A-V) Junctional Arrhythmias	112–129
8	Atrioventricular (A-V) Conduction Disturbances	130–144
9	Ventricular Arrhythmias	145–154
10	Intraventricular Conduction Disturbances	155–167
11	Wolff-Parkinson-White (WPW) Syndrome	168–176
12	Arrhythmias Related to Artificial Pacemakers	177–191
13	Miscellaneous	192–200

Suggested Reading

Index

Preface

Since 1972, when the first volume of this book was published, extensive investigative studies have been carried out in the fields of artificial cardiac pacing, the Wolff-Parkinson-White syndrome, and hemiblocks, bifascicular block and trifascicular block. Thus, a new chapter on the Wolff-Parkinson-White syndrome is added and the chapters dealing with artificial cardiac pacemakers and various intraventricular conduction disturbances have been significantly expanded.

In addition, a new chapter entitled "Normal Variants" is added for better understanding of various abnormal electrocardiograms. The section on electrolyte imbalance (Ch. 13, Miscellaneous) has also been markedly expanded.

Volume II presents 200 electrocardiographic tracings, each with a short case history to aid in the interpretation of the electrocardiogram. The aims and the basic designs of Volume II are essentially the same as those of Volume I. The unique feature of these volumes is the practical approach with clinical applications. The reverse side of each page gives a full analysis of the tracing so that each reader can assess his or her diagnosis. Arrows and various labels are used whenever applicable on the reversed side to help explain complicated electrocardiographic tracings. In the majority of cases, three simultaneous leads (leads V_1 II and V_5, or leads I, II and III) recorded by three-channel ECG equipment are shown for accurate diagnosis. In addition to the electrocardiographic diagnosis, the pertinent facts of clinical significance and the therapeutic approach are often included.

The arrangement of the text and illustrations is based upon the author's experience in teaching medical students, coronary care unit nurses and physicians with various backgrounds. This book is intended as a companion volume to the first volume; although the areas of study in this volume are basically the same as those of Volume I, none of the cases included here appear in the earlier volume.

The author hopes that the book will be of particular value to all medical students, house staff, cardiology fellows, and primary physicians including family physicians, emergency room physicians, internists and cardiologists. In addition, coronary care unit nurses, of course, will learn various electrocardiographic abnormalities, in great detail, by reading this book.

The secretarial burden was carried out cheerfully by Miss Theresa McAnally, personal secretary to the author. Her most able and devoted assistance and efforts have been certainly indispensable in the completion of this book. Finally, the endless cooperation of Harper and Row Publishers is greatly appreciated.

Edward K. Chung, M.D.

King of Prussia, Pennsylvania
January 1, 1977

ECG diagnosis
Self Assessment
Volume II

chapter 1
NORMAL VARIANTS

CASE 1

This electrocardiogram was obtained from a 65-year-old man with no demonstrable heart disease during his annual checkup. He was not taking any drug.

What is your ECG diagnosis?

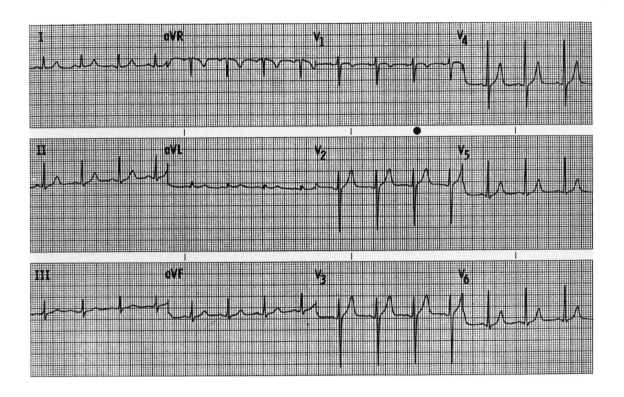

CASE 1: DIAGNOSIS

The cardiac rhythm is sinus with a rate of 90 beats per minute. The electrocardiogram is within normal limits.

The diagnostic criteria of normal sinus rhythm include:

1. P wave of sinus origin (P axis between 0 and $+90°$).
2. Constant P-P cycles (the shortest and the longest P-P intervals vary less than 0.16 second).
3. Normal P-R interval (between 0.12–0.20 second).
4. Constant P-R interval and each P wave followed by a QRS complex.
5. Atrial rate between 60–100 beats per minute.

In order to satisfy the above criteria, the P waves must be upright in lead II, whereas they should be inverted in lead aVR. The remaining limb leads (leads I, III, aVL, and aVF) may show various P wave configurations depending on the P axis. The P wave in lead V_1 (often V_2 as well) usually shows biphasic (positive component followed by negative component) configuration. The positive component of the P wave represents the right atrial depolarization while the negative component is due to the left atrial depolarization.

In the typical normal electrocardiogram as shown in this tracing, the amplitude of the R wave increases progressively from lead V_1 to V_6, but the actual R wave amplitude in leads V_4 through V_6 are similar in many instances. In fact, lead V_4 often exhibits the tallest R wave. The transitional QRS complex (RS complex) is commonly observed around lead V_3 or V_4.

The T waves in a normal ECG are upright in most limb leads, except for lead aVR, and all precordial leads. Lead V_1 may show upright, inverted, or biphasic T wave in normal individuals.

CASE 2

This electrocardiogram was obtained from an 18-year-old healthy woman during a routine physical checkup.

What is your ECG diagnosis?

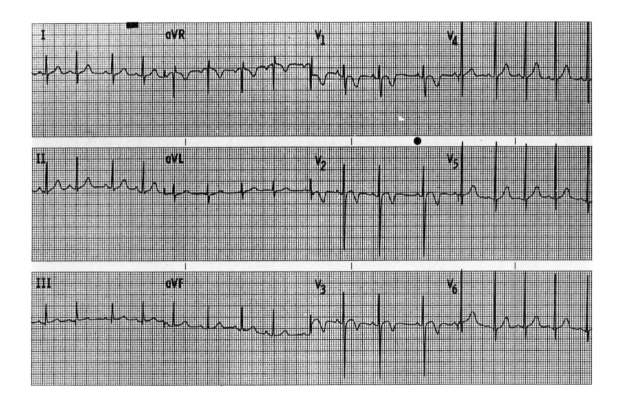

CASE 2: DIAGNOSIS

The cardiac rhythm is sinus arrhythmia with rate ranging from 83–100 beats per minute. It is obvious that the T waves are inverted in leads V_1 through V_3. This ECG finding is called "juvenile wave pattern" which is a normal variant in young individuals. The juvenile T wave change most commonly involves leads V_1 through V_3, and it seems to be more common in young females than males. The juvenile T wave pattern may be observed not uncommonly up to age 30, but at times, the juvenile T wave pattern may persist even in older adults, especially in women. When the juvenile T wave pattern is seen in older adults, it is difficult to distinguish from other ECG abnormalities such as myocardial ischemia or pulmonary embolism.

The juvenile T wave pattern is most commonly seen until late adolescence, and there is no racial difference regarding its incidence. The exact cause of the juvenile T wave pattern is not certain.

CASE 3

A 35-year-old black male was seen in the emergency room because of "indigestion."

What is your ECG diagnosis?

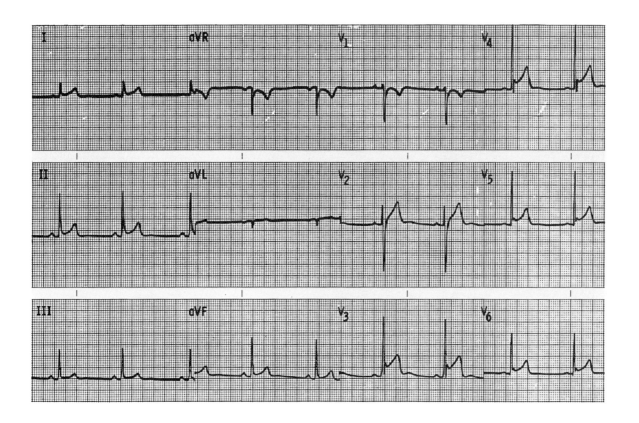

CASE 3: DIAGNOSIS

The cardiac rhythm is sinus bradycardia with a rate of 52 beats per minute. It is noteworthy that there is significant S-T segment elevation in many leads, more pronounced in the left precordial leads. This ECG finding has been called "early repolarization pattern" which is a normal variant.

The early repolarization pattern is most commonly encountered among young, black males (age between 15–40), and the finding, of course, has no clinical significance. The "J-point" is usually elevated in the early repolarization pattern, and the finding superficially resembles pericarditis (see Chapter 4) or myocardial injury (see Chapter 3).

The exact mechanism responsible for the production of so-called early repolarization pattern is not clearly understood.

Sinus bradycardia is not uncommon in healthy individuals.

CASE 4

This electrocardiogram was obtained from a 3-month-old girl with mild fever.

What is your ECG diagnosis?

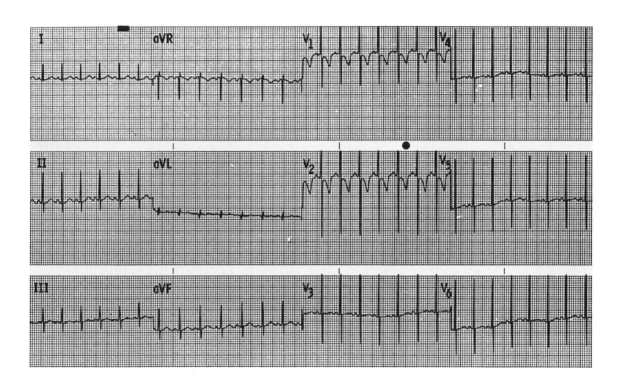

CASE 4: DIAGNOSIS

The cardiac rhythm is marked sinus tachycardia with a rate of 175 beats per minute. The R wave in lead V_1 is relatively tall (R:S ratio 1:1), and this is a normal finding in children. In addition, the juvenile T wave pattern (inverted T waves in leads V_1 and V_2) in this tracing is again a normal variant (see Case 2).

The heart rate is faster than usual for her age because marked sinus tachycardia is common during febrile illness in children.

In summary, the electrocardiographic findings in this case are within normal limits.

CASE 5

A 12-year-old girl was seen at the Pediatric Clinic during an annual checkup.

What is your ECG diagnosis?

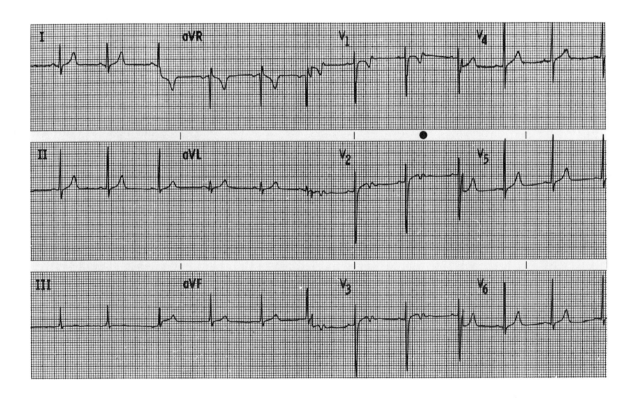

CASE 5: DIAGNOSIS

The cardiac rhythm is sinus arrhythmia with a rate of 70 beats per minute. It is interesting to note that the T waves are biphasic and irregular in shape in leads V_1 through V_3. This ECG finding is another example of the juvenile T wave pattern (see Case 2).

In most cases, the T waves are inverted (not deeply or symmetrically) in leads V_1 through V_3 (at times up to leads V_4 through V_6) in the juvenile T wave pattern (see Case 2), but occasionally, the T wave configuration may show a biphasic or irregular pattern.

This girl was found to be perfectly healthy, and the ECG finding is also within normal limits.

CASE 6

This ECG tracing was taken during a routine annual checkup on a 26-year-old healthy physician as part of a physical fitness program.

What is your ECG diagnosis?

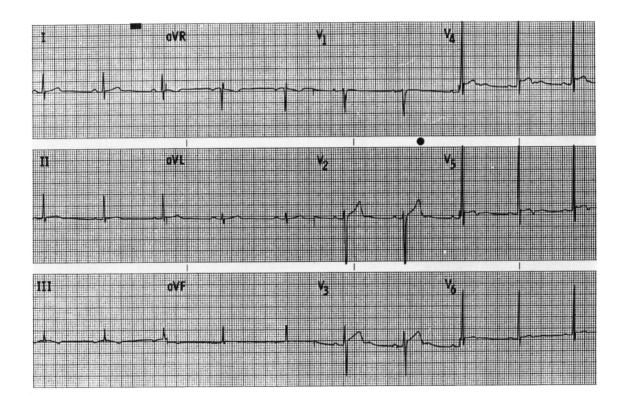

CASE 6: DIAGNOSIS

The cardiac rhythm is sinus bradycardia with a rate of 55 beats per minute. It is obvious that the T waves in leads V_4 through V_6 are either biphasic, inverted, or low in amplitude. This ECG finding is a rather unusual form of the juvenile T wave pattern (see Case 2). As indicated previously, the typical juvenile T wave pattern reveals inverted T waves primarily involving leads V_1 through V_3 (see Case 2).

It has been demonstrated that the atypical juvenile T wave pattern as shown in this case is observed almost always in extremely healthy, athletic young males. Again, the exact cause is uncertain, but it is known that this atypical juvenile T wave pattern is an unusual normal variant.

The ECG finding superficially simulates left ventricular hypertrophy (see Chapter 2), myocardial ischemia (see Chapter 3), or pericarditis (see Chapter 4). This young physician has been very athletic all his life.

CASE 7

This electrocardiogram was taken at the Psychiatric Service from a 40-year-old woman with a psychoneurotic disorder.

What is your ECG diagnosis?

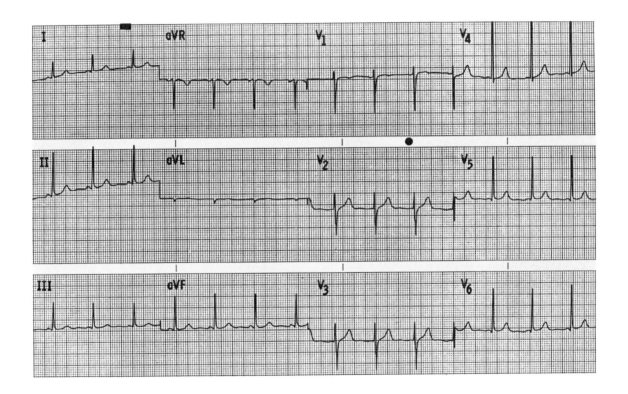

CASE 7: DIAGNOSIS

The basic rhythm is sinus with a rate of 82 beats per minute. It is noteworthy that the P-R interval is unusually short (P-R interval 0.08 second).

The short P-R interval is relatively common among patients with psychoneurotic disorders, individuals with anxiety, and any person during stressful situations. Thus, the short P-R interval is not uncommon during preoperative or postoperative periods, acute myocardial infarction, and before and after cardiac catheterization. In addition, the short P-R interval is a rather common finding in various high output states such as fever, anemia, and hyperthyroidism.

Whenever the P-R interval is short, on the other hand, a possibility of the Wolff–Parkinson–White syndrome, Lown–Ganong–Levine syndrome, or so-called coronary nodal rhythm can be raised (see Chapters 7 and 11).

In summary, the ECG finding in this case is a normal variant.

CASE 8

This electrocardiogram was obtained from a 26-year-old obese woman without demonstrable heart disease.

What is your ECG diagnosis?

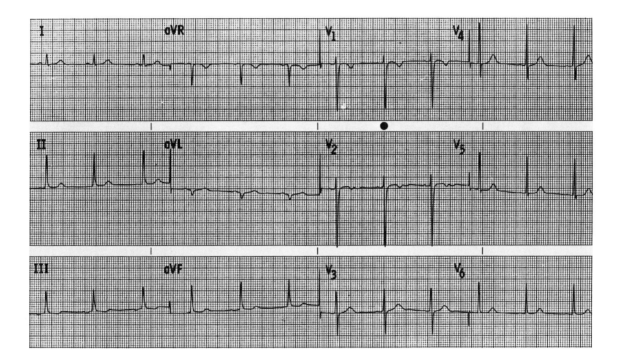

CASE 8: DIAGNOSIS

The cardiac rhythm is *not* typical sinus rhythm because the P axis is −30°. As described earlier, the P axis in the typical normal sinus rhythm is between 0 and +90° (see Case 1). In this case, the rhythm diagnosis is sinus rhythm with left axis deviation of the P waves.

It has been shown that the left axis deviation of the P waves may be encountered in obese individuals, as seen in this case, pregnant women, and patients with ascites or abdominal tumors. On the other hand, the left axis deviation of the P waves may be an early finding of left atrial enlargement. On rare occasions, left axis deviation of the P waves is seen in normal persons with no apparent cause.

In addition, there is juvenile T wave pattern (see Case 2). In summary, the electrocardiographic finding in this case is within normal limits.

CASE 9

A slender 19-year-old female college student was seen at the student health clinic for a routine checkup.

What is your ECG diagnosis?

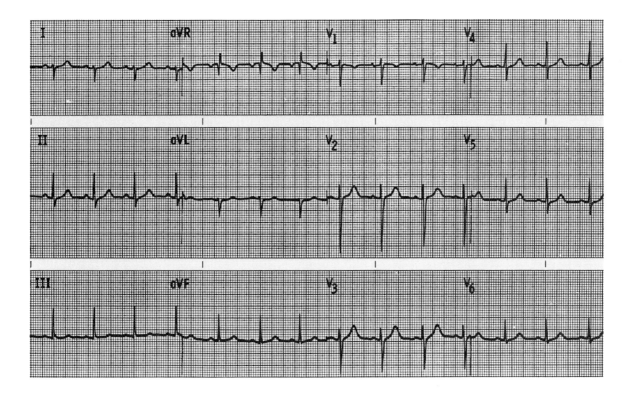

CASE 9: DIAGNOSIS

The cardiac rhythm is sinus with a rate of 84 beats per minute. The striking ECG finding in this tracing is right axis deviation of the QRS complexes (QRS axis +120°).

In slender individuals, as seen in this case, right axis deviation of the QRS complexes is not uncommon, and the finding is clinically insignificant.

On the other hand, two main possible causes for right axis deviation of the QRS complexes should always be considered. Namely, the right axis deviation of the QRS complexes may be due to right ventricular hypertrophy (see Chapter 2), or the finding may represent left posterior hemiblock (see Chapter 10).

In summary, the electrocardiographic finding in this case is a normal variant.

chapter 2
CHAMBER ENLARGEMENT (HYPERTROPHY)

CASE 10

This electrocardiogram was obtained from a 57-year-old female with hypertensive heart disease.

What is your ECG diagnosis?

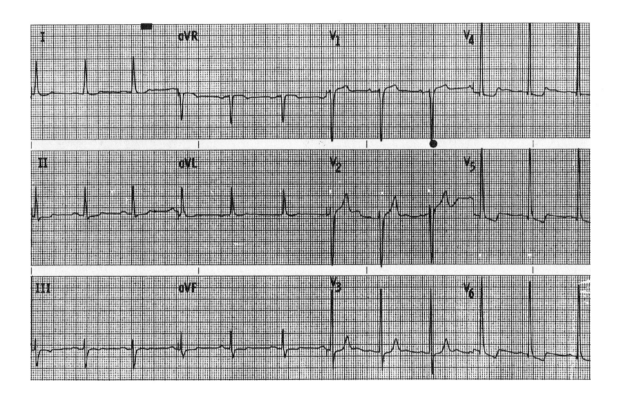

CASE 10: DIAGNOSIS

The cardiac rhythm is sinus with a rate of 68 beats per minute. The striking abnormality is markedly increased left ventricular force (tall R waves in leads V_4 through V_6 with deep S wave in lead V_1) associated with secondary S-T, T wave changes in leads V_4 through V_6. Thus, this tracing is a typical example of left ventricular hypertrophy (systolic overloading pattern).

The diagnostic criteria of left ventricular hypertrophy include:

1. Tall R wave in lead V_5 or $V_6 \geqq 26$ mm.
2. S wave in lead V_1 plus R wave in lead V_5 or $V_6 \geqq 35$ mm.
3. R wave in lead I $\geqq 15$ mm.
4. R wave in lead I plus S wave in lead III $\geqq 25$ mm.
5. R wave in lead aVL $\geqq 13$ mm.
6. Secondary S-T, T wave changes in leads I, aVL, and V_4 through V_6.

Among the above criteria, no. six with no. one or two are the most reliable findings in left ventricular hypertrophy. When the ECG findings meet the criteria of left ventricular hypertrophy but there is no S-T, T wave change, the finding may be due to diastolic overloading left ventricular hypertrophy such as is seen in aortic insufficiency (see Case 14). On the other hand, increased left ventricular voltage alone is often a normal finding in young, healthy individuals.

It is important to remember that left axis deviation of the QRS complexes in the limb leads is *not* a criterion for the diagnosis of left ventricular hypertrophy. At most, only less than 50% of left ventricular hypertrophy may show some degree of left axis deviation of the QRS complexes.

In addition to left ventricular hypertrophy, left atrial hypertrophy is suggested (notched and broad P waves in some limb leads).

It should be noted that the most common cause of left ventricular hypertrophy (systolic overloading pattern) is systemic hypertension. The next most common cause is aortic stenosis.

CASE 11

This ECG tracing was obtained from a 39-year-old man with aortic stenosis.

What is your ECG diagnosis?

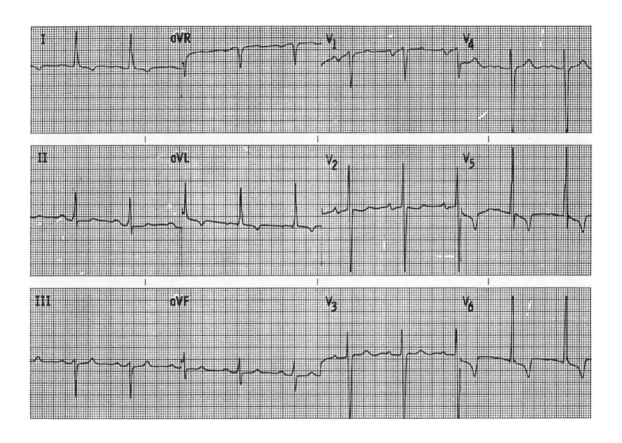

CASE 11: DIAGNOSIS

The rhythm is sinus (rate 64 beats per minute) with first degree A-V block (P-R interval 0.24 second). Utilizing the diagnostic criteria described in Case 10, the obvious diagnosis is left ventricular hypertrophy (systolic overloading pattern).

In addition, left atrial hypertrophy is also present. Whenever there is marked left ventricular hypertrophy either due to systemic hypertension or aortic stenosis, the left atrium is also significantly enlarged in most cases.

Diagnostic criteria of left atrial hypertrophy:

1. Broad (often notched) P waves in one or more limb leads (commonly in leads I, II, and aVL) $\geqq$ 3 mm.
2. Deep and broad negative component of P waves in leads V_1 and $V_2 \geqq$ 1 mm in depth and width.
3. Coarse atrial fibrillation waves $\geqq$ 1 mm in amplitude.

CASE 12

This electrocardiogram was obtained from a 53-year-old man who has been taking digoxin (0.25 mg) daily.

1. *What is your ECG diagnosis?*
2. *What is the most likely underlying heart disease?*

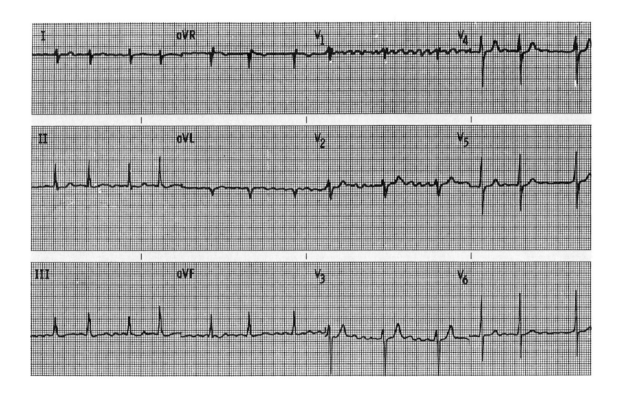

CASE 12: DIAGNOSIS

The cardiac rhythm is coarse atrial fibrillation with ventricular rate ranging from 64–95 beats per minute.

The diagnosis of right ventricular hypertrophy can be made without any difficulty on the basis of right axis deviation of the QRS complexes (QRS +105°) and relatively tall R waves (incomplete right bundle branch block pattern) in lead V_1. In addition, left atrial hypertrophy is also present because of coarse atrial fibrillation (see Case 11).

The diagnostic criteria of right ventricular hypertrophy include:

1. Right axis deviation of the QRS complexes with tall or relatively tall R wave (R:S ratio $\geqq$ 1) in lead V_1.
2. Right axis deviation with posterior axis deviation of the QRS complexes.
3. Right axis deviation of the QRS complexes with incomplete right bundle branch block pattern in lead V_1.
4. Secondary S-T, T wave changes in leads V_1 through V_3 (not essential).

When the ECG findings consist of coarse atrial fibrillation and right ventricular hypertrophy, the underlying heart disease is nearly always mitral stenosis.

CASE 13

This ECG tracing was obtained from a 73-year-old man who has been taking digoxin (0.25 mg) and hydrochlorothiazide (50 mg) daily for chronic congestive heart failure due to hypertensive heart disease.

What is your ECG diagnosis?

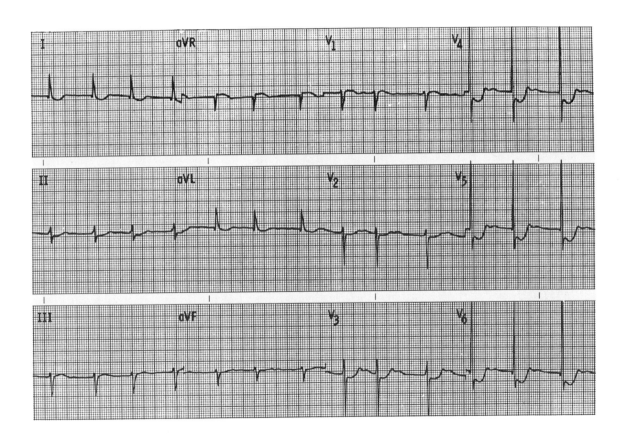

CASE 13: DIAGNOSIS

The underlying cardiac rhythm is atrial fibrillation with ventricular rate ranging from 70–83 beats per minute (see Chapter 6).

The diagnosis of left ventricular hypertrophy is obvious on the basis of tall R waves in leads V_4 through V_6 with the secondary S-T, T wave changes (see Case 10). The S-T segment depression may be partially due to digitalis effect.

In addition, prominent U waves (pronounced in leads V_2 through V_6) represent hypokalemia (see Chapter 13).

CASE 14

This electrocardiogram was obtained from a 41-year-old man with rheumatic aortic insufficiency. He was not taking any drug.

What is your ECG diagnosis?

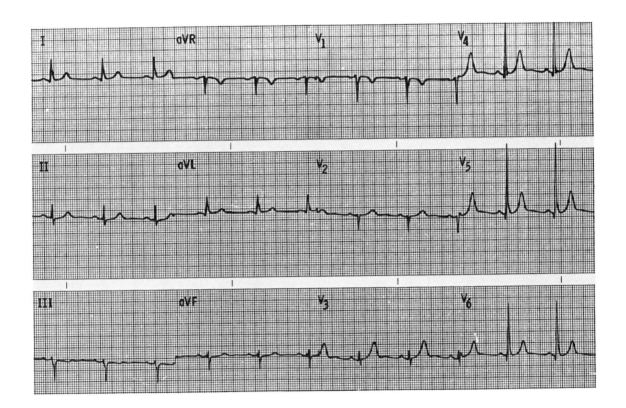

CASE 14: DIAGNOSIS

The cardiac rhythm is sinus with a rate of 65 beats per minute. The ECG tracing appears to be within normal limits, but the R wave amplitude in the left precordial leads is increased. Namely, diastolic overloading left ventricular hypertrophy is responsible for the tall R waves in leads V_4 through V_6. The T waves are normal (upright) in the left precordial leads in diastolic overloading left ventricular hypertrophy. Systolic overloading left ventricular hypertrophy is shown in Cases 10, 11, and 13, and the diagnostic criteria have been described previously (see Case 10).

It should be reemphasized that the high left ventricular voltage is relatively common in healthy, young individuals in many cases. Therefore, the ECG interpretation should be made according to the given clinical impression.

CASE 15

A 4-year-old boy was admitted to the Pediatric Cardiology Service for the evaluation of heart murmur.

1. *What is your ECG diagnosis?*
2. *What is the most likely underlying cardiac lesion?*

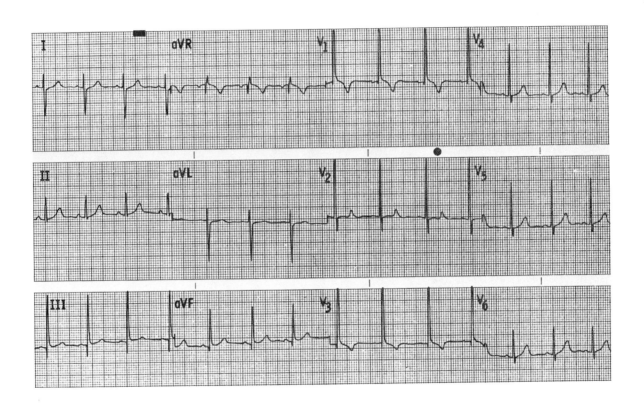

CASE 15: DIAGNOSIS

The cardiac rhythm is sinus arrhythmia with rate ranging from 75–85 beats per minute.

The diagnosis of right ventricular hypertrophy is obvious on the basis of right axis deviation (QRS axis +120°) of the QRS complexes and tall R waves in leads V_1 through V_3 with the secondary S-T, T wave changes (see Case 12). In severe right ventricular hypertrophy, a small q wave in lead V_1 (sometimes up to leads V_2 and V_3) is not uncommon. This is considered to be a result of altered initial septal activation due to marked right ventricular hypertrophy.

When lead V_1 (often leads V_2 and V_3 as well) shows a very tall R wave with or without a small q wave due to right ventricular hypertrophy in children, the underlying lesion is most commonly congenital pulmonic stenosis, which this boy has.

CASE 16

This electrocardiogram was obtained from a 62-year-old man with rheumatic heart disease, and he has been taking digoxin (0.25 mg) and hydrochlorothiazide (50 mg) daily.

1. *What is your ECG diagnosis?*
2. *What is the most likely underlying valvular lesion?*

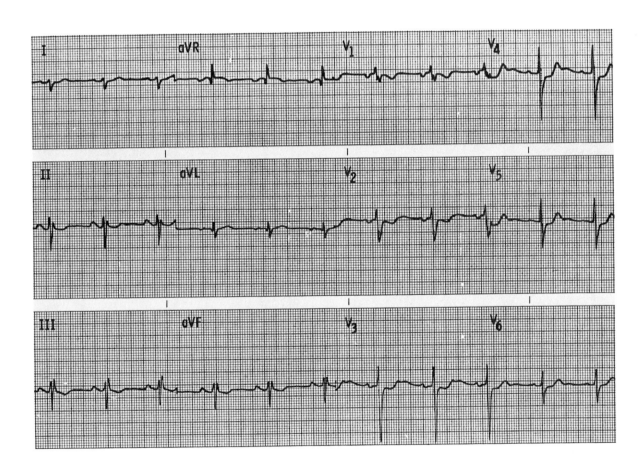

CASE 16: DIAGNOSIS

The cardiac rhythm is sinus with a rate of 67 beats per minute. The diagnosis of right ventricular hypertrophy can be made on the basis of right axis deviation of the QRS complexes (QRS axis $+240°$) and relatively tall R wave (incomplete right bundle branch block pattern) in lead V_1 (see Case 12). In addition, broad and notched P waves in limb leads with deep and wide negative component of the P waves in leads V_1 and V_2 represent left atrial hypertrophy (P-mitrale, see Case 11).

Furthermore, hypokalemia is diagnosed because of prominent U waves, especially in leads V_2 and V_3 (see Chapter 13). The S-T segment depression in many leads represents digitalis effect.

When the ECG abnormalities consist of right ventricular hypertrophy and left atrial hypertrophy (P-mitrale), the underlying lesion is usually mitral stenosis. In right ventricular hypertrophy in mitral stenosis, the R wave in lead V_1 is not extremely tall, and the QRS configuration often shows atypical incomplete right bundle branch block pattern or RS pattern in lead V_1.

CASE 17

This ECG tracing was obtained from a 56-year-old man with rheumatic heart disease. He has been taking digoxin (0.25 mg) daily.

1. *What is your ECG diagnosis?*
2. *What is the most likely underlying valvular lesion?*

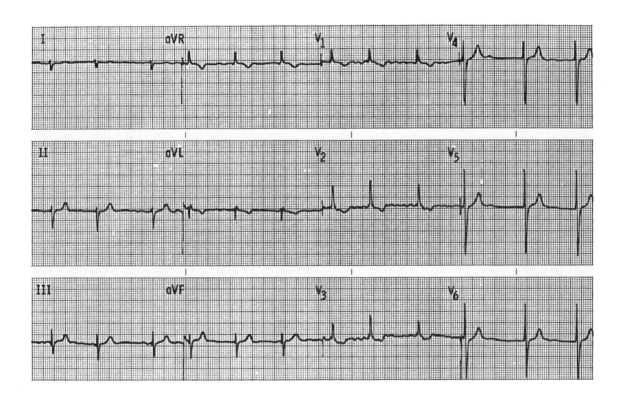

CASE 17: DIAGNOSIS

The cardiac rhythm is coarse atrial fibrillation with ventricular rate ranging from 60–80 beats per minute.

The diagnosis of right ventricular hypertrophy can be made without any difficulty on the basis of right axis deviation of the QRS complexes (QRS axis +210°) and tall R waves in leads V_1 through V_3 associated with secondary S-T, T wave changes. Coarse atrial fibrillation represents left atrial hypertrophy.

The diagnosis of mitral stenosis is almost certain when the ECG abnormalities consist of right ventricular hypertrophy and coarse atrial fibrillation (see also Cases 12 and 16).

CASE 18

A 59-year-old woman was admitted to the hospital because of advanced congestive heart failure.

  1. What is your ECG diagnosis?
  2. What is the most likely underlying disorder?

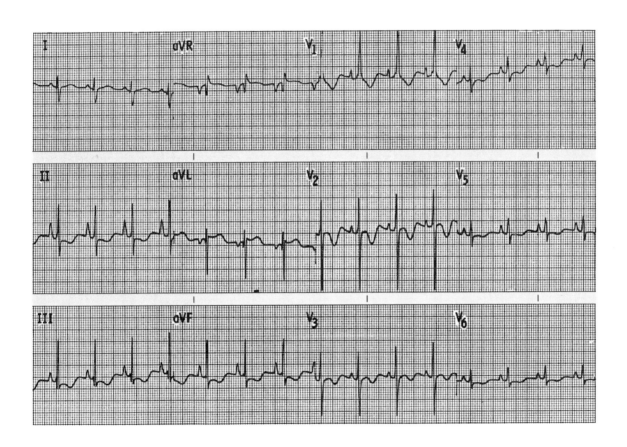

CASE 18: DIAGNOSIS

Cardiac rhythm is sinus with a rate of 94 beats per minute. Marked right ventricular hypertrophy is diagnosed on the basis of a tall R wave in lead V_1 and right axis deviation of the QRS complexes (QRS axis $+120°$) associated with secondary S-T, T wave changes in leads V_1 through V_3 (see Case 12).

Another striking ECG abnormality is peaked and tall P waves in leads II, III, aVF, and many precordial leads. This ECG finding represents right atrial hypertrophy. Right atrial hypertrophy due to pulmonary disease is termed "P-pulmonale," whereas right atrial hypertrophy in congenital heart disease is called "P-congenitale" as seen in pulmonic stenosis, Ebstein's anomaly and atrial septal defect.

The diagnostic criteria of right hypertrophy include:

1. Peaked and tall P waves in leads II, III, and aVF $\geqq 3$ mm.
2. Peaked and tall P waves in leads V_1 and $V_2 \geqq 2$ mm.

Needless to say, this patient has been suffering from a long-standing obstructive pulmonary disease leading to chronic cor-pulmonale.

CASE 19

This electrocardiogram was obtained from a 24-year-old man with chronic pulmonary disease associated with kyphosclerosis.

What is your ECG diagnosis?

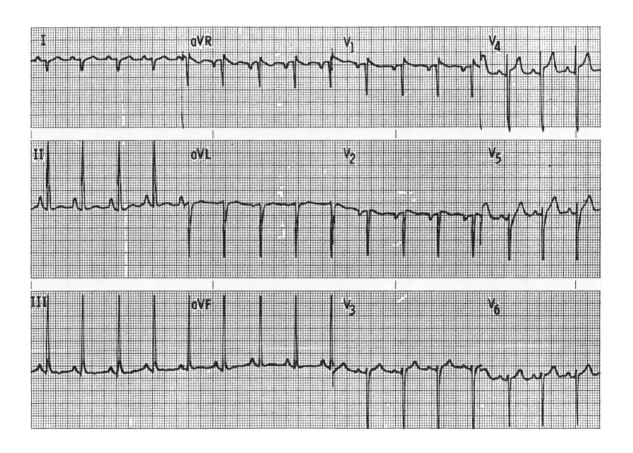

CASE 19: DIAGNOSIS

The underlying cardiac rhythm is sinus tachycardia with a rate of 103 beats per minute.

A combination of right axis deviation (QRS axis +105°) with posterior axis deviation of the QRS complexes is diagnostic of right ventricular hypertrophy (see Case 12). Right ventricular hypertrophy consisting of right axis and posterior axis deviation is almost always due to either chronic cor-pulmonale or mitral stenosis.

Another ECG finding is P-pulmonale which represents right atrial hypertrophy (see Case 18).

It is important to recognize that a pseudo-anteroseptal myocardial infarction pattern is produced in this case because of marked posterior axis deviation of the QRS complexes.

CASE 20

This ECG tracing was obtained postoperatively from a 10-year-old girl with transposition of the great vessels. This slow cardiac rhythm associated with congestive heart failure persisted postoperatively.

1. *What is your cardiac rhythm diagnosis?*
2. *What is your ECG diagnosis?*
3. *What is the treatment of choice?*

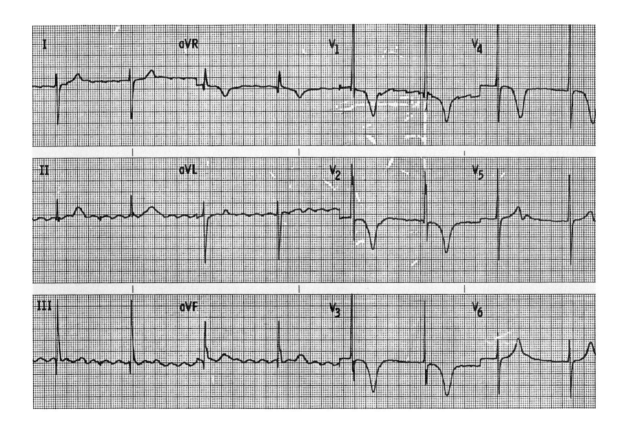

CASE 20: DIAGNOSIS

Cardiac rhythm reveals atrial flutter (atrial rate 265 beats per minute) with A-V junctional escape rhythm (ventricular rate 45 beats per minute) due to complete A-V block (see Chapter 8).

There is marked right ventricular hypertrophy on the basis of tall R wave in lead V_1 with right axis deviation of the QRS complexes (QRS axis $+135°$).

The treatment of choice for symptomatic complete A-V block is permanent artificial pacemaker implantation.

In general, when the A-V ratio appears to be more than 5:1 in atrial flutter and the ventricular cycles are regular, complete A-V block is most likely present. Complete A-V block is confirmed in this case when the F-R distance (distance from the last flutter wave to the next QRS complex) varies throughout the tracing.

The inverted T waves in leads V_1 through V_4 in this tracing are due to a combination of juvenile T wave pattern (see Case 2) and right ventricular hypertrophy (see Case 12).

CASE 21

A 49-year-old man was admitted to the Coronary Care Unit because of severe congestive heart failure.

    1. What is your ECG diagnosis?
    2. What is the most likely underlying disorder?

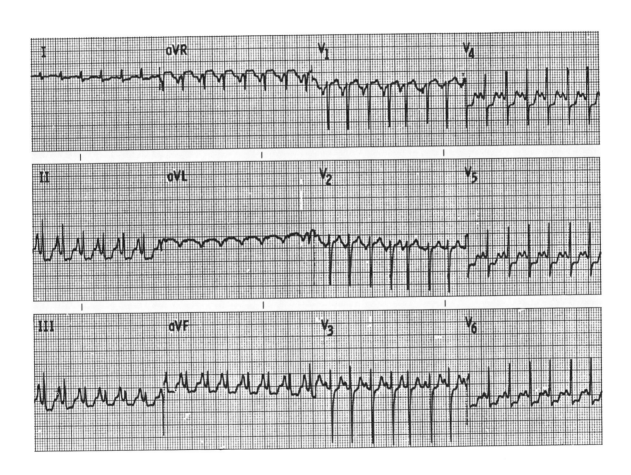

CASE 21: DIAGNOSIS

The rhythm is marked sinus tachycardia with a rate of 175 beats per minute and an atrial premature contraction (19th beat).

The P waves are extremely peaked and tall because of P-pulmonale (right atrial hypertrophy). In addition, S-T segment depression is noted in many leads, and this finding represents diffuse subendocardial injury which is at least partially due to the very rapid rate.

The underlying disorder is chronic cor-pulmonale due to obstructive pulmonary disease.

He was digitalized rapidly in conjunction with the treatment of the underlying pulmonary disease.

CASE 22

This electrocardiogram was obtained from a 31-year-old woman with rheumatic heart disease. She has been taking digoxin (0.25 mg) daily.

What is your ECG diagnosis?

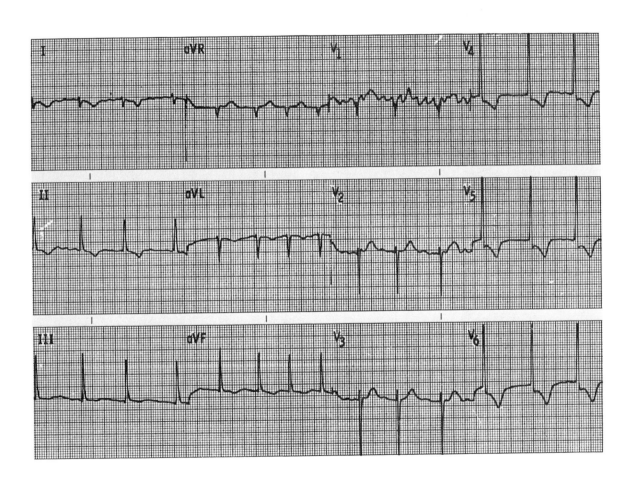

CASE 22: DIAGNOSIS

Cardiac rhythm reveals coarse atrial fibrillation with ventricular rate ranging from 75–100 beats per minute.

The ECG findings in the precordial leads are diagnostic of left ventricular hypertrophy (see Case 10). However, the right axis deviation of the QRS complexes (QRS axis +100°) in the limb leads is incompatible with a pure left ventricular hypertrophy; the right axis deviation is due to right ventricular hypertrophy. Thus, this patient has evidences of biventricular hypertrophy.

In addition, coarse atrial fibrillation is indicative of left atrial hypertrophy (see Case 11).

This patient was found to have multivalvular lesions including mitral stenosis and mitral insufficiency, as well as aortic stenosis. She underwent cardiac surgery for mitral and aortic valve replacement.

CASE 23

This electrocardiogram was obtained from a 53-year-old man with rheumatic heart disease. Digitalis toxicity was suspected.

What is your ECG diagnosis?

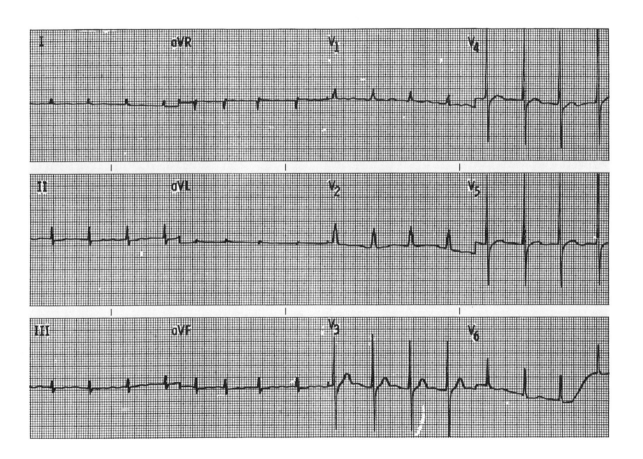

CASE 23: DIAGNOSIS

This ECG finding represents intermittent nonparoxysmal A-V junctional tachycardia with a rate of The underlying cardiac rhythm is atrial fibrillation, but the R-R intervals are regular in many areas. 93 beats per minute.

Nonparoxysmal A-V junctional tachycardia, particularly in the presence of pre-existing atrial fibrillation, is probably the most common digitalis-induced arrhythmia.

It should be noted that the R waves are primarily upright in all precordial leads, with high amplitude in leads V_4 and V_5. These findings most likely represent biventricular hypertrophy.

This patient was found to have mitral stenosis as well as mitral insufficiency.

Silght S-T segment depression in some leads is indicative of digitalis effect.

CASE 24

This ECG tracing was obtained from a 2-month-old boy with congestive heart failure due to patent ductus arteriosus. He has been digitalized.

What is your ECG diagnosis?

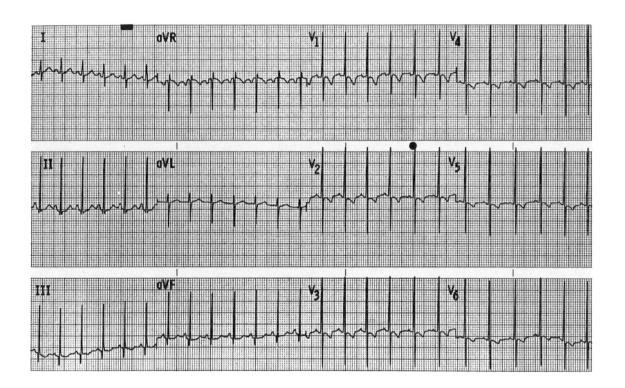

CASE 24: DIAGNOSIS

The rhythm is sinus tachycardia with a rate of 132–160 beats per minute.

The R waves are tall practically in all precoridal leads, and this ECG finding is diagnostic for biventricular hypertrophy. The diagnosis of biventricular hypertrophy is further supported by the "Katz–Wachtel phenomenon" (large voltage of equiphasic QRS complexes in the mid-precordial leads).

The electrocardiogram is often normal in mild cases of patent ductus arteriosus. Left ventricular hypertrophy with a diastolic overloading pattern (see Case 14) is usually produced with a large defect. In severe cases, especially associated with significant pulmonary hypertension, biventricular hypertrophy may develop as seen in this boy. Left atrial hypertrophy and first degree A-V block are not uncommon, and right bundle branch block may be encountered occasionally.

Diffuse S-T, T wave changes may be due to biventricular hypertrophy itself and/or digitalis effect.

CASE 25

This electrocardiogram was obtained from a 50-year-old man with aortic stenosis and coronary heart disease.

What is your ECG diagnosis?

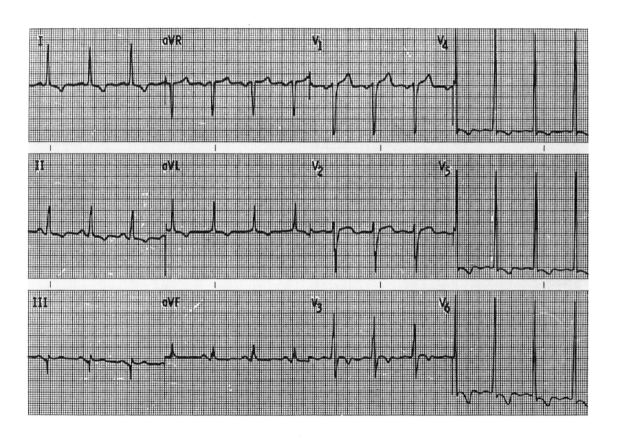

CASE 25: DIAGNOSIS

The cardiac rhythm is sinus with a rate of 82 beats per minute. The diagnosis of left ventricular hypertrophy is obvious on the basis of extremely tall R waves in leads V_4 through V_6 with secondary S-T, T wave changes and deep S wave in lead V_1 (see Case 10). In addition, left atrial enlargement is also suggested because of deep and broad negative component of the P wave in lead V_1 (see Case 11).

Another ECG abnormality is Q wave in leads III and aVF strongly suggestive of old diaphragmatic (inferior) myocardial infarction.

CASE 26

This electrocardiogram was obtained from a 76-year-old man with hypertensive and coronary heart disease.

What is your ECG diagnosis?

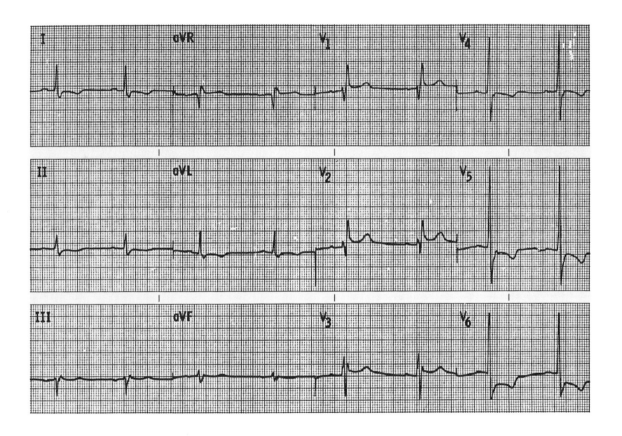

CASE 26: DIAGNOSIS

The cardiac rhythm is marked sinus bradycardia with a rate of 48 beats per minute.

It is readily recognized that there is evidence of left ventricular hypertrophy (see Case 10). Another ECG abnormality is right bundle branch block diagnosed on the basis of RR' (M shape) of the QRS configuration in leads V_1 through V_3, with slurred S waves in leads I, aVL, and V_4 through V_6.

In addition, there is another ECG finding in this tracing. Namely, the S-T segment elevation with upright T waves in leads V_1 through V_3 are *not* due to a pure right bundle branch block. These ECG findings represent coexisting myocardial ischemia and injury (see Chapter 3).

This patient has been suffering from angina pectoris for several years. Marked sinus bradycardia in this case was induced by propranolol (Inderal) which was prescribed for angina pectoris and hypertension.

CASE 27

A 23-year-old woman was admitted to the Cardiac Service for the evaluation of her cardiac status.

1. *What is your ECG diagnosis?*
2. *What is the most likely underlying heart disease?*

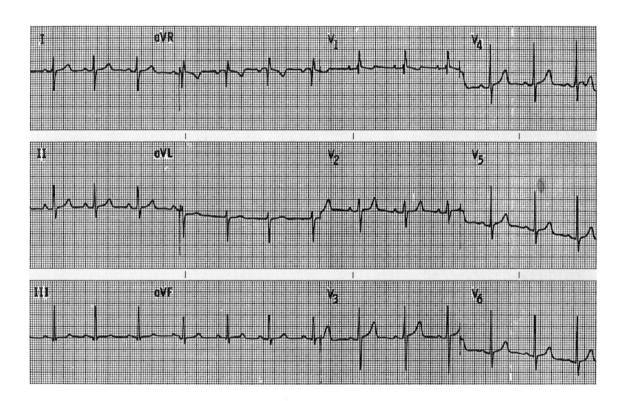

CASE 27: DIAGNOSIS

The cardiac rhythm is sinus with a rate of 78 beats per minute.

The striking ECG abnormality is incomplete right bundle branch block *pattern* with right axis deviation of the QRS complexes (QRS axis +105°) suggestive of right ventricular hypertrophy.

When dealing with this type of ECG abnormality in young individuals, the underlying heart disease is nearly always atrial septal defect, which this patient has.

Right bundle branch block (either complete or incomplete) *pattern* is almost always found (up to 90–95%) in cases with all types of atrial septal defect. Incomplete right bundle branch block *pattern* is more common, as seen in this case, than the complete right bundle branch block. Right bundle branch block *pattern* has been attributed to hypertrophy of the crista supraventricularies rather than to a true right bundle branch block.

The QRS axis in atrial septal defect, secundum type, is frequently right axis deviation because of right ventricular hypertrophy with a diastolic overloading pattern, but the QRS axis may be normal. Ostium primum defect usually produces left axis deviation in the presence of right bundle branch block. Under this circumstance, the left axis deviation is considered to represent congenital left anterior hemiblock (see Chapter 10).

chapter 3

MYOCARDIAL ISCHEMIA, INJURY, AND INFARCTION

CASE 28

A 60-year-old hypertensive man was admitted to the Coronary Care Unit because of exertional chest pain.

What is your ECG diagnosis?

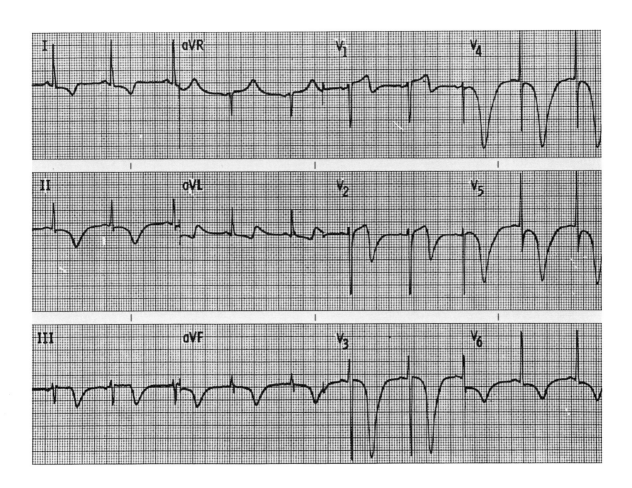

CASE 28: DIAGNOSIS

The cardiac rhythm is sinus with a rate of 63 beats per minute.

Deeply and symmetrically inverted T waves are recognizable in practically all leads. This ECG finding represents diffuse myocardial ischemia. By determining serial serum enzyme studies, SGOT, CPK, and LDH levels were reported to be within normal limits. In addition, serial electrocardiograms failed to show any evidence of acute myocardial infarction.

In addition to diffuse myocardial ischemia, the diagnosis of left ventricular hypertrophy can be made with certainty (see Case 10).

It has been suggested that subendocardial infarction should be strongly considered if the symmetrically and deeply inverted T waves persist more than a week. The term "giant T wave syndrome," has been applied when the T waves are deeply and symmetrically inverted as seen in this case.

CASE 29

A 78-year-old man with known coronary heart disease was admitted to the Coronary Care Unit because of increasing severity of chest pain associated with palpitations.

1. What is your ECG diagnosis?
2. What is the treatment of choice?

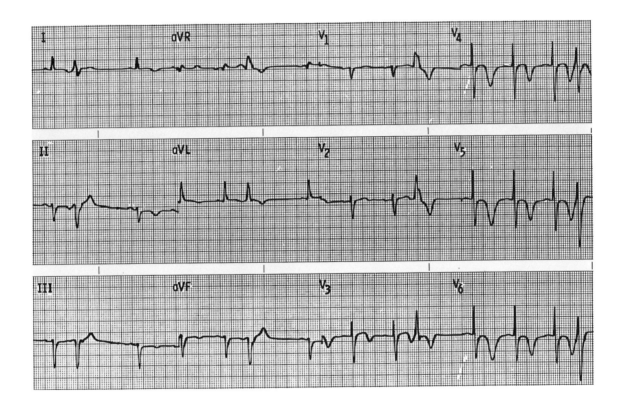

CASE 29: DIAGNOSIS

The basic cardiac rhythm is sinus with a rate of 78 beats per minute. In addition, there are frequent ventricular premature contractions producing ventricular quadrigeminy. It is extremely important to note that the coupling interval (the interval from the ectopic beat to the preceding beat of the basic rhythm) is very short so that the T wave of the preceding beat is partially interrupted. This finding is called the "R-on-T phenomenon." It has been repeatedly documented that the threshold for the initiation of ventricular fibrillation is very low during a vulnerable period (the R-on-T phenomenon) of the ventricle (corresponding to the top of the T wave). This is more so during an acute coronary event.

The T waves are symmetrically inverted practically in all leads indicative of diffuse myocardial ischemia. In addition, left anterior hemiblock is diagnosed on the basis of marked left axis deviation of the QRS complexes (QRS axis −60°, see Chapter 10).

The treatment of choice for the ventricular premature contractions in acute coronary event is intravenous injection of lidocaine (Xylocaine).

Regarding the management of ventricular arrhythmias, the treatment is considered to be indicated in the following situations:

1. Frequent (6 or more per minute) ventricular premature contractions.
2. Multifocal ventricular premature contractions.
3. R-on-T phenomenon.
4. Ventricular groups beats.
5. Paroxysmal ventricular tachycardia.
6. Ventricular flutter or fibrillation.
7. Exercise-induced ventricular arrhythmias.

CASE 30

A 50-year-old man was referred to the Cardiology Service for the evaluation of chest pain of several weeks' duration.

The 12-lead ECG shown on this page was taken at rest as a control tracing. On the reverse page, the exercise (treadmill) ECG test is shown.

1. *What is your ECG diagnosis of the tracing shown on this page?*
2. *What is the result of the exercise ECG test shown on the next page?*

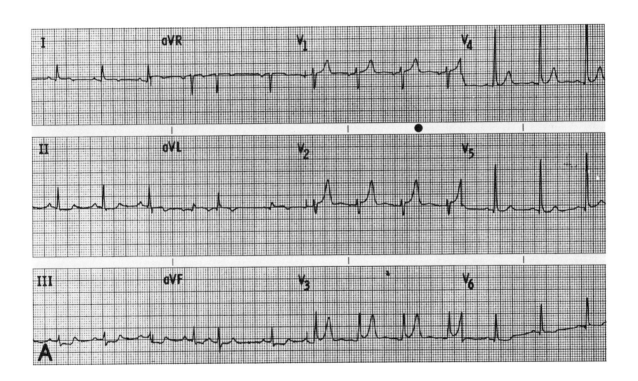

CASE 30: DIAGNOSIS

The 12-lead ECG (shown on the reveres page) shows sinus rhythm (rate 78 beats per minute) and an atrial premature contraction with aberrant ventricular conduction (fifth beat).

Posterior myocardial ischemia is strongly suggested on the basis of tall T waves in leads V_1 through V_3. In addition, the S-T segment is slightly depressed in leads II, III, aVF, and V_6 compatible with diaphragmatic-lateral subendocardial injury.

The exercise (treadmill) ECG test was recorded by using a two-channel ECG recorder (leads II and V_5). Rhythm strip A was taken at rest, whereas strips B and C were recorded during exercise. Strips D to F were obtained at a 1-minute interval following termination of an exercise. The exercise was terminated prematurely because of severe chest pain associated with significant S-T segment depression and frequent ventricular premature contractions with groups beats.

The exercise ECG test is unequivocally positive in this patient.

He underwent coronary arteriography followed by coronary bypass surgery with marked improvement.

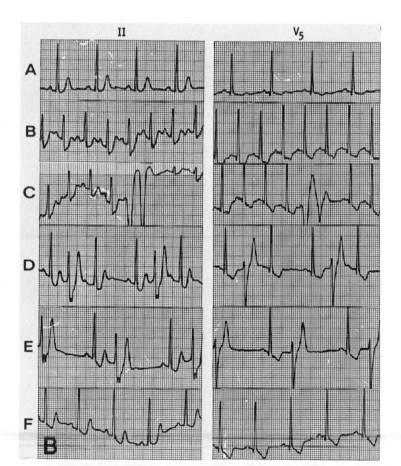

CASE 31

A 45-year-old woman was seen at the Cardiac Clinic for the evaluation of her chest pain. Exercise (treadmill) ECG test was performed.

What is the result of the exercise ECG test?

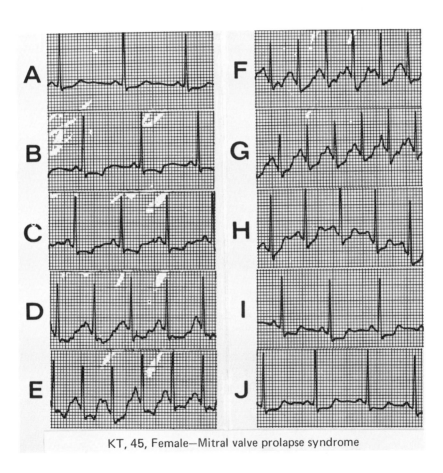

KT, 45, Female—Mitral valve prolapse syndrome

CASE 31: DIAGNOSIS

The exercise ECG rhythm strips represent lead V_5. Strips *A* and *B* were taken at rest in supine and standing positions, respectively. Strips *C* to *G* were recorded during exercise with a 2-minute interval, whereas strips *H* to *J* were obtained after exercise with a 1-minute interval.

There are marked S-T, T wave changes diagnostic for the positive exercise ECG test. However, she was found to have mitral valve prolapse syndrome confirmed by echocardiogram and cardiac catheterization. Coronary arteriogram failed to show any evidence of coronary artery disease.

Therefore, her exercise ECG test is considered to be a false positive test which is reported to be common in patients with mitral valve prolapse syndrome. Atypical chest pain is the most common presenting symptom of mitral valve prolapse syndrome.

CASE 32

A 79-year-old man was admitted to the Coronary Care Unit because of severe chest pain of 2–3 hours' duration.

What is your ECG diagnosis?

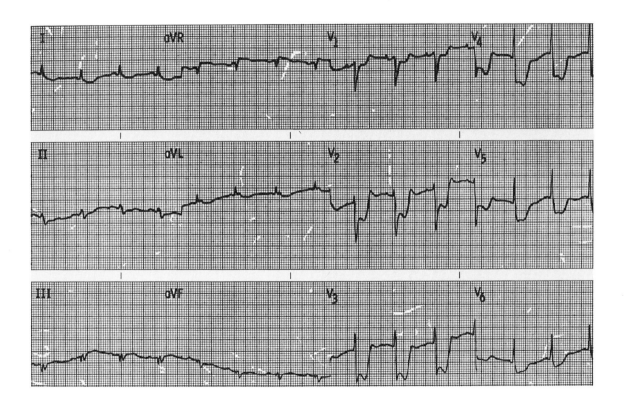

CASE 32: DIAGNOSIS

The cardiac rhythm is sinus with a rate of 87 beats per minute. It is easy to appreciate marked S-T segment depression in all precordial leads, particularly pronounced in leads V_2 through V_5. This ECG finding represents anterior subendocardial injury. Subendocardial infarction should be strongly considered when marked S-T segment depression persists more than a week. It should be remembered that no pathologic Q waves are produced in subendocardial infarction.

The QRS voltage is markedly diminished in limb leads. When the total sum of the QRS voltage (both positive and negative components) in leads I, II, and III is 15 mm or less, the term "low voltage" is used. Low voltage is very common in patients with acute coronary events. In addition, low voltage may be encountered in patients with pulmonary emphysema, obesity, myxedema, pleural effusion, pericardial effusion, acute congestive heart failure, and cardiomyopathy.

CASE 33

A 52-year-old man was admitted to the Coronary Care Unit because of chest pain. The ECG tracing shown on this page was taken during chest pain (tracing A), whereas the ECG tracing shown on the next page was obtained during a pain-free period (tracing B).

What is your ECG diagnosis?

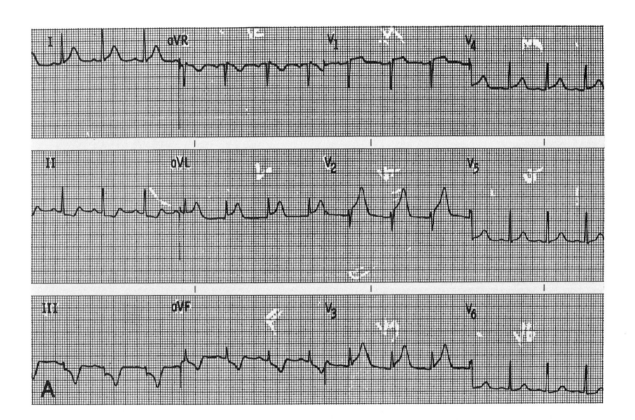

CASE 33: DIAGNOSIS

The cardiac rhythm of both tracings *A* and *B* is sinus with a rate of 80 beats per minute.

Tracing A shows S-T segment elevation in leads I, aVL, and V_1 through V_4, indicative of anterior subepicardial injury. Leads II, III, and aVF reveal S-T segment depression as a reciprocal change. It is interesting to note that tracing B is entirely within normal limits.

This type of angina pectoris has been termed "Prinzmetal's angina," "atypical angina," and "variant angina." Characteristic features of Prinzmetal's angina are that S-T segment elevation occurs only during chest pain, and the ECG tracing returns to normal as soon as the patient is free of chest pain. In addition, the angina attack is *not* exertional chest pain, and the pain is often unpredictable.

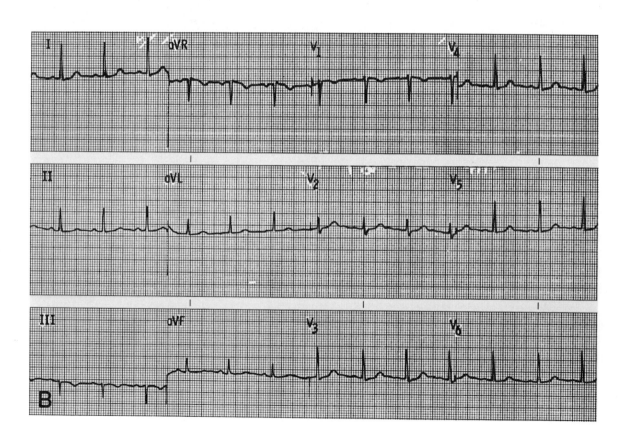

CASE 34

This electrocardiogram was obtained from a 56-year-old man with coronary heart disease and hypertensive heart disease. He has been taking propranolol (Inderal) (30 mg) four times daily for hypertension and chest pain.

What is your ECG diagnosis?

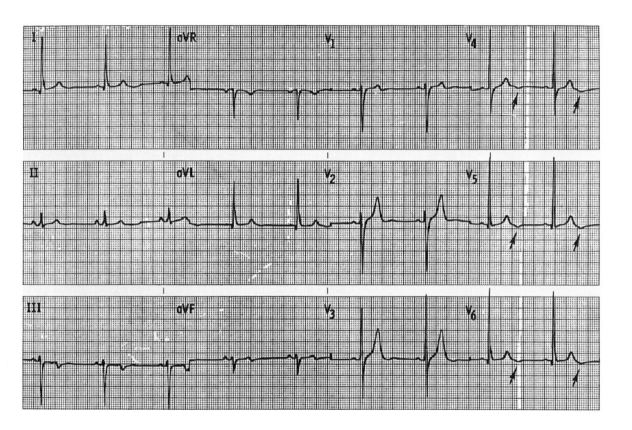

CASE 34: DIAGNOSIS

The cardiac rhythm is sinus bradycardia with a rate of 52 beats per minute. Left ventricular hypertrophy is suggested by voltage (see Case 10). It is not uncommon to observe that the T waves are often upright for some years in patients with proven left ventricular hypertrophy with mild hypertension.

Another interesting ECG finding in this tracing is inverted U waves (indicated by arrows) which usually represent myocardial ischemia In patients with angina pectoris. In addition, relatively tall T waves in leads V_1 through V_3 may represent posterior myocardial ischemia.

Sinus bradycardia in this patient is most likely due to propranolol (Inderal) effect.

CASE 35

A 50-year-old man was admitted to the Coronary Care Unit because of severe chest pain of a few hours' duration.

What is your ECG diagnosis?

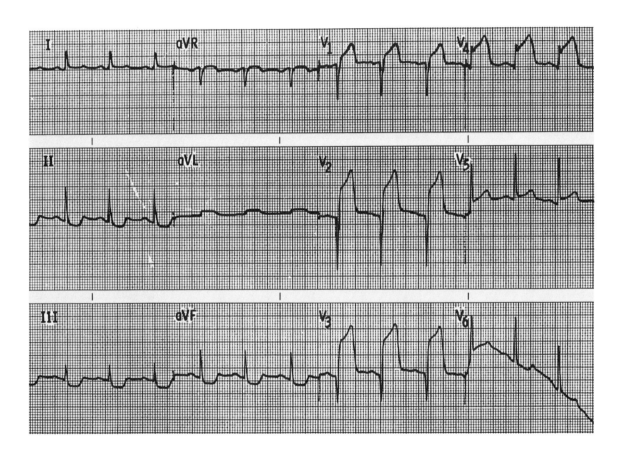

CASE 35: DIAGNOSIS

The cardiac rhythm is sinus with a rate of 84 beats per minute.

It is obvious that the S-T segment is markedly elevated in leads V_1 through V_4 with a loss of R waves (Q-S wave or Q wave). This ECG abnormality is unequivocal evidence of acute anteroseptal myocardinal infarction. The S-T segment depression in leads II, III, and aVF represent a reciprocal change.

When dealing with this type of ECG change, myocardial infarction is usually less than 12 hours (often 4–5 hours) old. The S-T segment elevation in leads facing the involved area is almost always markedly elevated in an early phase of acute myocardial infarction. The S-T segment elevation alone is termed subepicardial injury which has been commonly called "current injury."

CASE 36

This electrocardiogram was obtained from a 42-year-old man with coronary heart disease.

What is your ECG diagnosis?

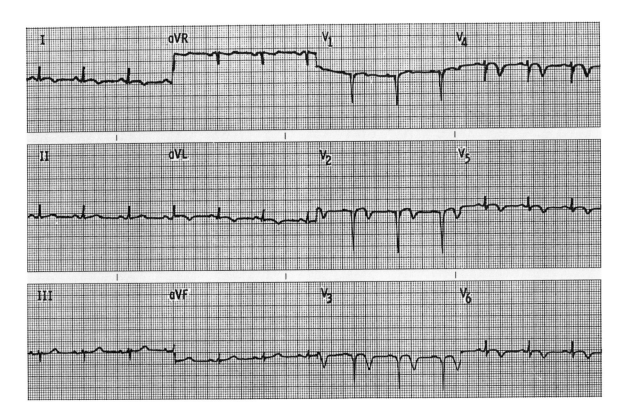

CASE 36: DIAGNOSIS

The cardiac rhythm is sinus with a rate of 75 beats per minute. There is a complete loss of R waves in leads V_1 through V_3 with inverted T waves in leads I, aVL, and V_1 through V_6. This ECG finding definitely represents anteroseptal myocardial infarction. However, it is impossible to determine the exact duration of myocardial infarction unless serial ECG tracings are available for comparison or clinical data are available. The reason for this is that the T wave inversion may last for 1 week to months or years and even indefinitely after myocardial infarction occurred. In other words, the age of myocardial infarction is uncertain when the S-T segment elevation is no longer present in a given tracing. In general, the S-T segment elevation (subepicardial injury) lasts not more than 1 week. When the S-T segment elevation lasts more than a week, ventricular aneurysm should be strongly considered.

By taking a careful history, this patient most likely had suffered from myocardial infarction 6 weeks previously.

The QRS complexes in limb leads show low amplitude (low voltage) which is common in patients with myocardial infarction.

CASE 37

This ECG tracing was obtained from an obese 32-year-old woman with previous history of "heart attack."

What is your ECG diagnosis?

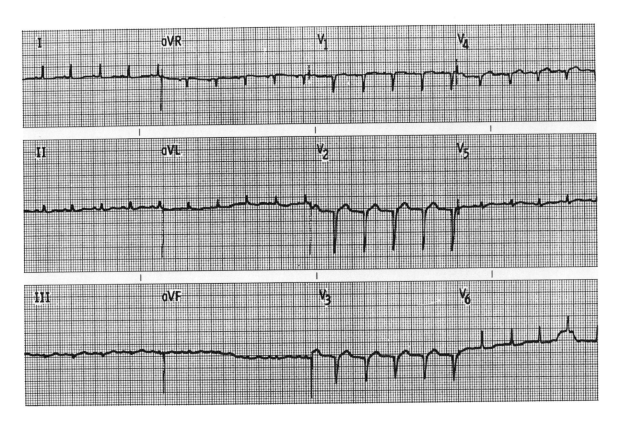

CASE 37: DIAGNOSIS

The cardiac rhythm reveals sinus tachycardia with a rate of 120 beats per minute.

Old anteroseptal myocardial infarction can be diagnosed without any difficulty on the basis of a loss of R waves in leads V_1 through V_3 with an embryonic R wave in lead V_4. Note that the T waves are upright in leads V_1 through V_4, and there is no S-T segment elevation.

In addition, markedly low voltage of the QRS complexes in many leads is due to two factors including myocardial infarction and obesity.

This patient had suffered from myocardial infarction 6 months previously. Obesity is, needless to say, the major contributing factor to cause myocardial infarction at a young age in this woman.

Other risk factors for premature atherosclerosis include hypertension, diabetes mellitus, hyperlipidemia, smoking, stress, etc., in addition to a genetic factor.

Sinus tachycardia with moderate degree (rate 110–125 beats per minute) is very common in obese individuals as seen in this case.

CASE 38

A 31-year-old obese and diabetic woman was admitted to the Coronary Care Unit because of severe chest pain of 2–3 hours' duration. The ECG tracing shown on this page was taken on admission (tracing A), while another ECG tracing shown on the next page was obtained a week later (tracing B).

What is your ECG diagnosis?

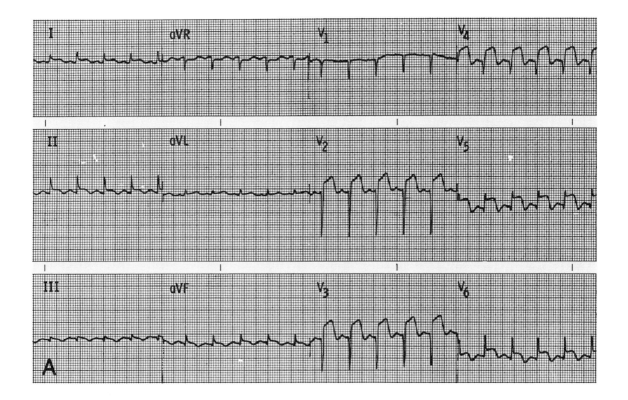

CASE 38: DIAGNOSIS

In tracing A, the cardiac rhythm is marked sinus tachycardia with a rate of 130 beats per minute. The diagnosis of acute extensive anterior myocardial infarction is readily made on the basis of marked S-T segment elevation with Q-S or Q waves in all precordial leads. In addition, acute diaphragmatic (inferior) myocardial infarction can be diagnosed on the basis of Q waves, S-T segment elevation and T wave inversion in leads II, III, and aVF.

Marked sinus tachycardia is extremely common during an early phase of acute myocardial infarction. Low voltage of the QRS complexes is due to her obesity and acute myocardial infarction.

The S-T segment elevation in many leads is much less pronounced in the ECG tracing taken 1 week later, but the T wave inversion is more evident (tracing B). The prolonged Q-T interval in acute ischemic event as seen in tracing B is extremely common in acute myocardial infarction.

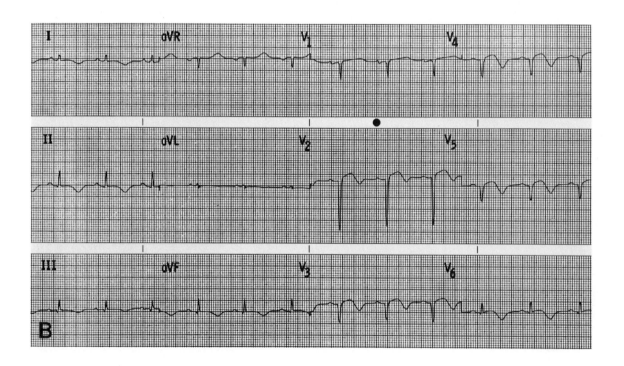

CASE 39

This electrocardiogram was obtained from a 71-year-old woman with coronary heart disease.

What is your ECG diagnosis?

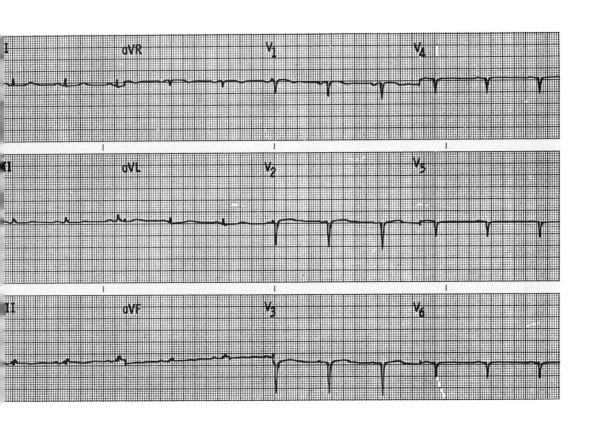

CASE 39: DIAGNOSIS

The cardiac rhythm is sinus with a rate of 65 beats per minute. Old extensive anterior myocardial infarction is diagnosed on the basis of Q-S waves in leads V_1 through V_5 with an embryonic R wave in lead V_6. The S-T segment is *not* elevated, and the T waves are biphasic or flat in all precordial leads. The biphasic or flat T waves are nonspecific abnormalities which are common in elderly individuals.

In addition, low voltage of the QRS complexes in limb leads is obvious in this tracing. The low voltage is common in elderly individuals and in patients with myocardial infarction. The low voltage has been described in detail previously (see Case 32).

This patient had suffered from myocardial infarction 1 year ago.

CASE 40

This ECG tracing was obtained from a 59-year-old woman with chronic congestive heart failure due to coronary heart disease. She had suffered from "heart attack" 6 months previously. She has been taking digoxin (0.125 mg) and hydrochlorothiazide (50 mg) daily.

What is your ECG diagnosis?

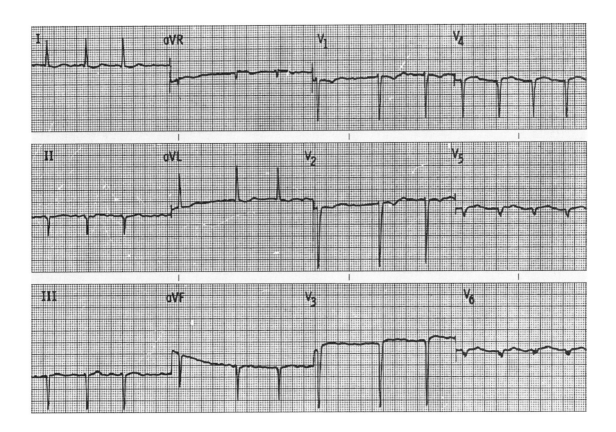

CASE 40: DIAGNOSIS

The cardiac rhythm reveals atrial fibrillation with rate ranging from 65–95 beats per minute. Old extensive anterior myocardial infarction can be diagnosed without any difficulty on the basis of embryonic R waves in leads V_1 and V_2 and Q-S waves in leads V_3 through V_6. In addition, the diagnosis of left anterior hemiblock is made because of marked left axis deviation (QRS axis $-50°$, see Chapter 10). Left ventricular hypertrophy is also suggested (see Case 10).

Another ECG abnormality is prominent U waves, suggestive of hypokalemia (see Chapter 13).

CASE 41

This electrocardiogram was obtained from a 53-year-old man with coronary heart disease. He was admitted to the Coronary Care Unit because of chest pain of 4–5 days' duration.

What is your ECG diagnosis?

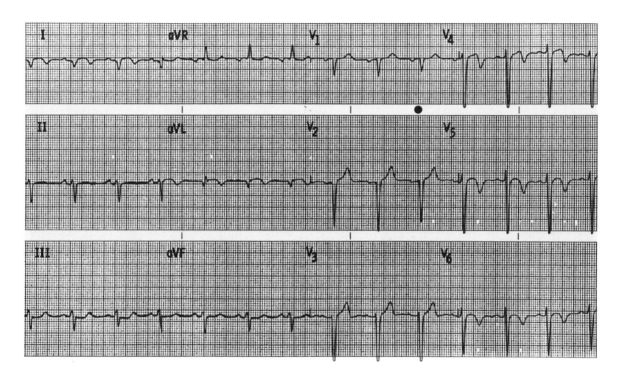

CASE 41: DIAGNOSIS

The cardiac rhythm is sinus with a rate of 78 beats per minute. High lateral myocardial infarction is diagnosed on the basis of Q-S waves in leads I and aVL associated with S-T segment elevation and T wave inversion. In addition, a localized anterior myocardial infarction can be diagnosed on the basis of a loss of R wave in lead V_2 (note that an embryonic R wave is present in lead V_1). The T waves are inverted in leads V_4 through V_6 because of lateral myocardial ischemia.

Another ECG abnormality in this tracing is left anterior hemiblock because of marked superior axis deviation. The typical features of left anterior hemiblock (see Chapter 10) are altered in this tracing because of a coexisting high lateral myocardial infarction; that is, the QRS axis is deviated superiorly and toward the right side instead of toward the left because of left anterior hemiblock plus high lateral myocardial infarction.

CASE 42

A 29-year-old diabetic man with strong family history of coronary heart disease was admitted to the Coronary Care Unit because of chest pain of 5–6 days' duration.

What is your ECG diagnosis?

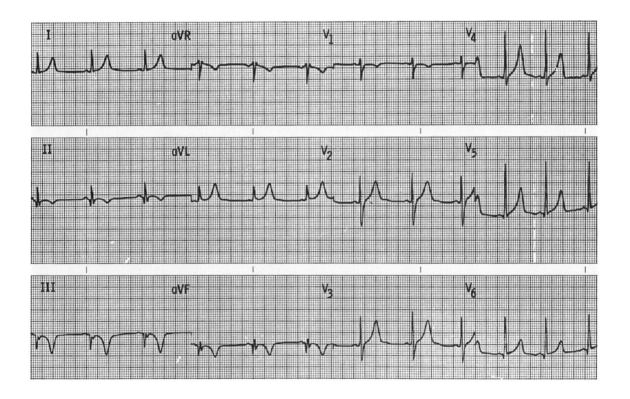

CASE 42: DIAGNOSIS

The cardiac rhythm is sinus arrhythmia with rate ranging from 62–80 beats per minute. Recent diaphragmatic (inferior) myocardial infarction is diagnosed on the basis of pathologic Q waves in leads II, III, and aVF with deeply and symmetrically inverted T waves.

It is noteworthy that the P-R interval is relatively short. As described previously (see Case 7), the short P-R interval is a common finding in any stressful situation such as is seen in acute myocardial infarction.

Diabetes mellitus and the genetic factor obviously contributed to the development of myocardial infarction at an early age in this case.

CASE 43

This electrocardiogram was obtained from a 65-year-old man with coronary heart disease.

What is your ECG diagnosis?

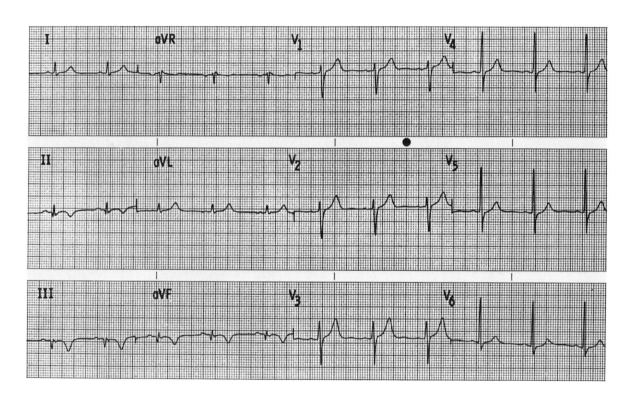

CASE 43: DIAGNOSIS

The cardiac rhythm is sinus with a rate of 67 beats per minute. The obvious diagnosis is recent diaphragmatic (inferior) myocardial infarction based on the pathologic Q waves in leads II, III, and aVF with deeply and symmetrically inverted T waves.

Another ECG abnormality in this tracing is relatively tall T waves in leads V_1 through V_3. This ECG finding most likely represents posterior myocardial ischemia. It has been shown that the T wave is biphasic or inverted in lead V_1 in the majority of healthy individuals above age 60. There is also a low voltage of the QRS complexes (see Case 32).

It has been well documented that diaphragmatic myocardial infarction and posterior myocardial ischemia frequently coexist.

CASE 44

A 48-year-old hypertensive and obese woman was admitted to the Coronary Care Unit because of a sharp chest pain of 6–7 hours' duration.

What is your ECG diagnosis?

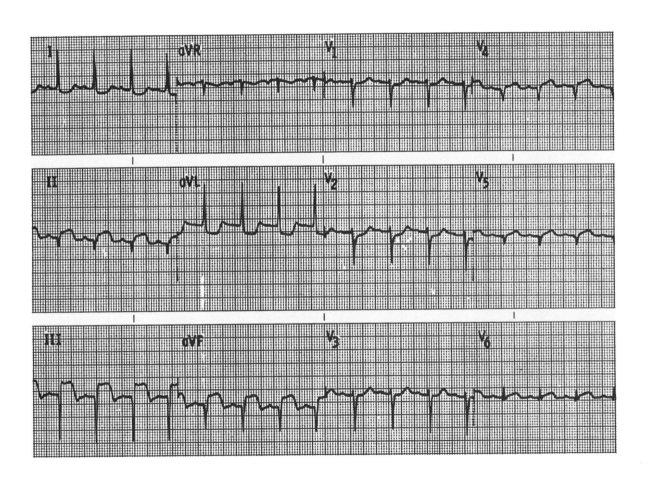

CASE 44: DIAGNOSIS

The cardiac rhythm is sinus tachycardia with a rate of 104 beats per minute.

The striking ECG abnormality is acute diaphragmatic (inferior) lateral myocardial infarction, Note a loss of the R waves in leads V_4 and V_5 with Q wave and markedly reduced R wave amplitude in lead V_6 representing lateral wall myocardial infarction.

In addition, left ventricular hypertrophy is strongly suggested on the basis of tall R waves in leads I and aVL, with deep Q-S wave in lead III (see Case 10). The typical features of left ventricular hypertrophy (see Case 10) is not shown in the precordial leads because of a coexisting lateral myocardial infarction.

It should be remembered that marked left axis deviation (QRS axis —45°) in this ECG tracing is a direct result of diaphragmatic myocardial infarction. Therefore, left axis deviation due to diaphragmatic myocardial infarction is actually a pseudo-left axis deviation. Needless to say, the diagnosis of left anterior hemiblock should not be made under this circumstance.

CASE 45

This electrocardiogram was obtained from a 32-year-old man with a strong family history of coronary heart disease. He was seen by a physician because of chest pain of recent onset.

What is your ECG diagnosis?

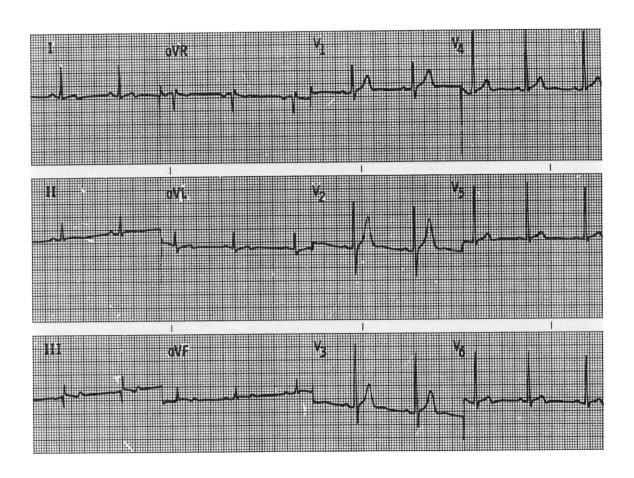

CASE 45: DIAGNOSIS

Cardiac rhythm is sinus with a rate of 65 beats per minute. It should be noted that the R wave as well as the T wave are tall in lead V_1. This ECG finding represents a true posterior myocardial infarction. In addition, the T waves are biphasic to inverted in leads I, III, aVL, aVF, and V_6. These T wave changes are most likely due to diaphragmatic lateral myocardial ischemia.

It should be stressed that no pathologic Q wave is produced in a true posterior myocardial infarction because there is no ECG lead facing the posterior wall. Actually, the tall R wave with tall T wave in lead V_1 is a reciprocal change of the pathologic Q wave with inverted T wave.

He was admitted to the Coronary Care Unit immediately. Coronary arteriography was performed followed by coronary bypass surgery with uneventful recovery.

CASE 46

A 68-year-old woman was admitted to the Coronary Care Unit because of severe chest pain of a few hours' duration.

What is your ECG diagnosis?

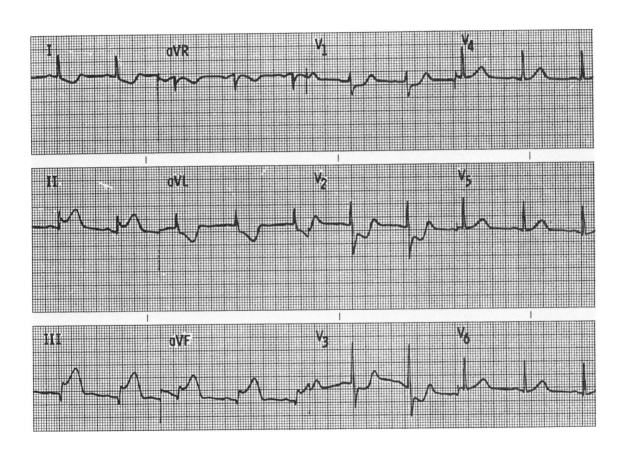

CASE 46: DIAGNOSIS

The caridac rhythm is sinus with a rate of 65 beats per minute.

The diagnosis of acute diaphragmatic (inferior) myocardial infarction can be made on the basis of pathologic Q waves in leads II, III, and aVF with marked S-T segment elevation in the same leads. The S-T segment depression in leads I and aVL represents a reciprocal change of acute diaphragmatic myocardial infarction.

In addition, acute true posterior myocardial infarction can be diagnosed because of relatively tall R wave in lead V_1 with S-T segment depression and upright T waves in leads V_1 through V_3.

Thus, a complete ECG diagnosis of this tracing is acute diaphragmatic (inferior)-posterior myocardial infarction.

CASE 47

This electrocardiogram was obtained from a 47-year-old man with chest pain of 1 week's duration.

What is your ECG diagnosis?

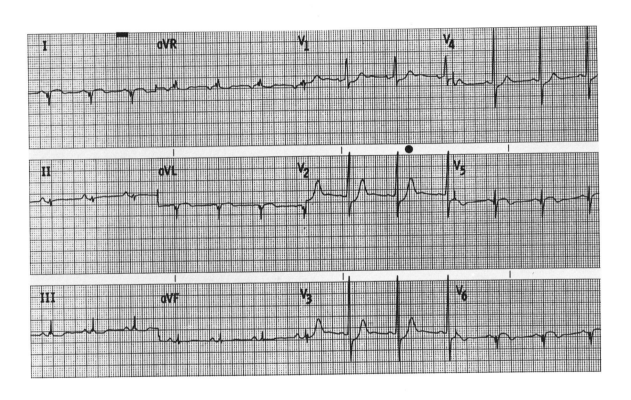

CASE 47: DIAGNOSIS

The cardiac rhythm is sinus with a rate of 78 beats per minute.

The striking ECG abnormality in this tracing is tall R waves in leads V_1 through V_3 with S-T segment depression and upright T waves in the same leads. These ECG findings represent a recent posterior myocardial infarction (see also Cases 45 and 46).

Another ECG abnormality is Q waves or Q-S waves in leads I, aVL, V_5 and V_6 with S-T segment elevation and T wave inversion. These findings are due to recent lateral myocardial infarction including high lateral wall involvement (changes in leads I and aVL).

A final ECG diagnosis of this tracing is recent posterolateral (including high lateral wall) myocardial infarction.

Note also a low voltage of the QRS complexes in the limb leads (see Case 32).

CASE 48

This ECG tracing was obtained from a 64-year-old man with coronary heart disease.

What is your ECG diagnosis?

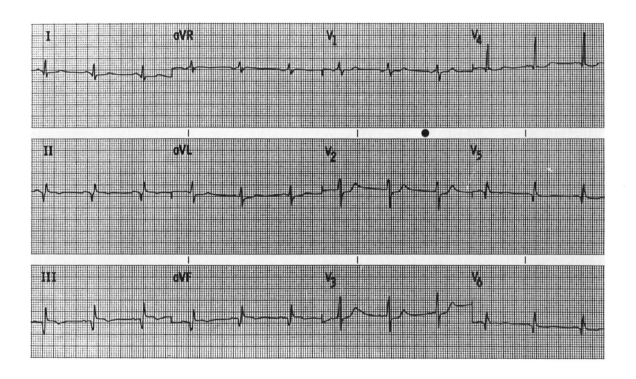

CASE 48: DIAGNOSIS

The cardiac rhythm is sinus with a rate of 70 beats per minute.

It should be noted that there are many leads showing pathologic Q waves with slight S-T segment elevation. Namely, myocardial infarction has occurred in the diaphragmatic (inferior) wall (Q waves in leads II, III, and aVF) as well as the lateral wall (Q waves in leads V_5 and V_6) including high lateral wall (Q waves in leads I and aVL).

Another ECG abnormality is a relatively tall R wave in lead V_1 with slight S-T segment depression in leads V_1 through V_3 as a result of a true posterior myocardial infarction.

Thus, a complete ECG diagnosis of this tracing is recent diaphragmatic (inferior) posterolateral myocardial infarction (DPLMI).

It has been shown that multiple (often triple) vessels are usually involved to produce DPLMI in most cases.

CASE 49

A 72-year-old woman was admitted to the Coronary Care Unit because of severe chest pain associated with cardiogenic shock. She expired within 48 hours as a result of myocardial rupture (proven by a postmortem examination).

What is your ECG diagnosis?

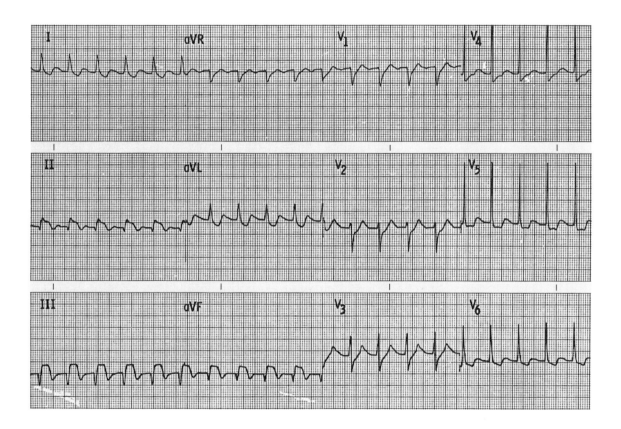

CASE 49: DIAGNOSIS

The cardiac rhythm reveals sinus tachycardia with a rate of 120 beats per minute.

Acute diaphragmatic (inferior) myocardial infarction can be diagnosed without any difficulty on the basis of pathologic Q waves in leads II, III, and aVF with S-T segment elevation and T wave inversion in the same leads. In addition, posterior subepicardial injury with ischemia can be suspected because of the S-T segemnt depression with upright T waves in leads V_1 through V_3.

Another ECG abnormality is left ventricular hypertrophy (see Case 10).

In general, the prognosis is not favorable when sinus tachycardia persists in patients with acute myocardial infarction. The underlying causes for the persisting sinus tachycardia may include cardiogenic shock, congestive heart failure, pulmonary embolism, extension of acute myocardial infarction, myocardial rupture, and bronchopneumonia, etc.

CASE 50

A 76-year-old hypertensive man was admitted to the Coronary Care Unit because of chest pain.

What is your ECG diagnosis?

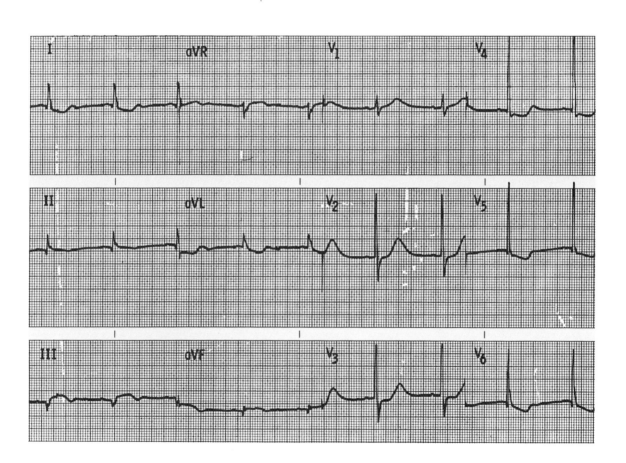

CASE 50: DIAGNOSIS

The cardiac rhythm is sinus bradycardia with a rate of 55 beats per minute.

The diagnosis of recent diaphragmatic (inferior) myocardial infarction can be established without any difficulty on the basis of abnormal Q waves in leads II, III, and aVF with S-T segment elevation and T wave inversion in the same leads. In addition, recent posterior myocardial infarction is diagnosed because of relatively tall R waves in lead V_1 with upright T waves and S-T segment depression in leads V_1 through V_3.

Another ECG abnormality is systolic over-loading left ventricular hypertrophy (see Case 10), as a result of systemic hypertension.

Thus, a complete ECG diagnosis of this tracing is recent diaphragmatic-posterior myocardial infarction associated with left ventricular hypertrophy. Sinus bradycardia is very common in recent diaphragmatic myocardial infarction.

CASE 51

This electrocardiogram was obtained from a 59-year-old man with coronary heart disease. He developed chest pain very recently, and his electrocardiogram taken 1 week prior to admission was said to be unremarkable. There was no history of fainting episodes.

1. What is your ECG diagnosis?
2. Is artificial pacing indicated?

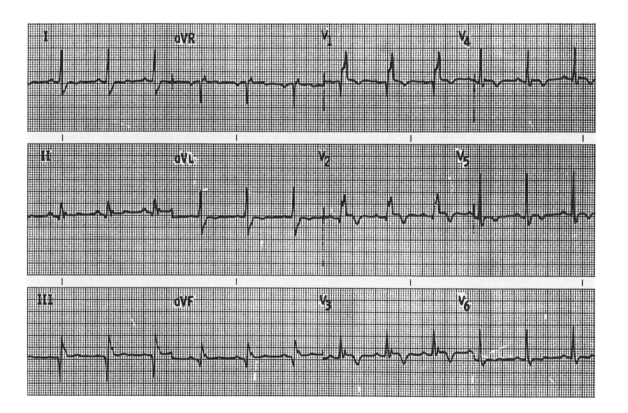

CASE 51: DIAGNOSIS

The cardiac rhythm is sinus with a rate of 75 beats per minute.

The diagnosis of recent diaphragmatic myocardial infarction is obvious because of abnormal Q waves in leads II, III, and aVF with S-T segment elevation.

Another striking ECG abnormality is right bundle branch block (see Chapter 10). With close observation, however, it can be recognized that the Q waves in leads V_1 and V_2 with S-T segment elevation and T wave inversion in all precordial leads are *not* due to right bundle branch block. Rather, there is definite evidence of recent anteroseptal myocardial infarction with diffuse anterior myocardial ischemia. In fact, this patient developed right bundle branch block secondary to anteroseptal myocardial infarction.

It is generally agreed that the prophylactic artificial pacing is considered to be *not* indicated for right bundle branch block due to anterior myocardial infarction.

A complete ECG diagnosis of this tracing is, therefore, recent diaphragmatic and anteroseptal myocardial infarction with diffuse anterior myocardial ischemia associated with right bundle branch block.

CASE 52

This electrocardiogram was obtained from a 69-year-old man with coronary heart disease.

What is your ECG diagnosis?

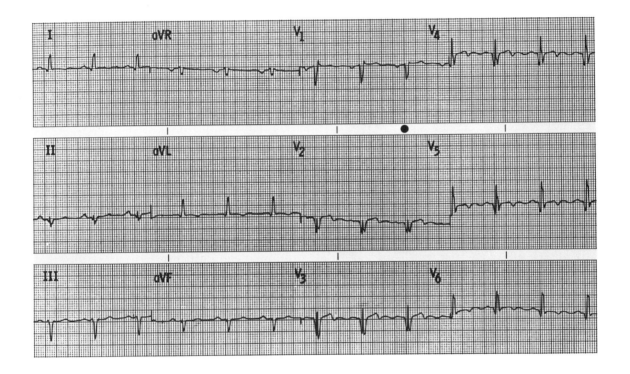

CASE 52: DIAGNOSIS

The cardiac rhythm is sinus with a rate of 76 beats per minute. There are pathologic (abnormal) Q waves in practically all precordial leads except for lead V_1, which shows an embryonic R wave. This ECG finding represents extensive anterior myocardial infarction including high lateral wall (Q waves in lead I and aVL). The exact duration of the myocardial infarction is uncertain because there are inverted T waves in leads V_2 through V_5 without significant S-T segment elevation. When dealing with this kind of ECG tracing, myocardial infarction could be anywhere between 1 week to many years old, because the T wave inversion may last weeks, months, or even years after myocardial infarction. In addition, old diaphragmatic myocardial infarction is a good possibility (Q wave or Q-S wave in leads II and aVF).

It should be noted that the QRS interval is broad, particularly in the precordial leads. This ECG finding is called "diffuse or nonspecific intraventricular block" which is not due to right or left bundle branch block (see Chapter 10). Diffuse intraventricular block is not uncommon in patients with extensive (massive) myocardial infarction. Some investigators use the term "intramyocardial block" to designate this finding.

CASE 53

This ECG tracing was obtained from an 86-year-old man approximately 2 weeks after the occurrence of his "heart attack." He developed intractable congestive heart failure.

What is your ECG diagnosis?

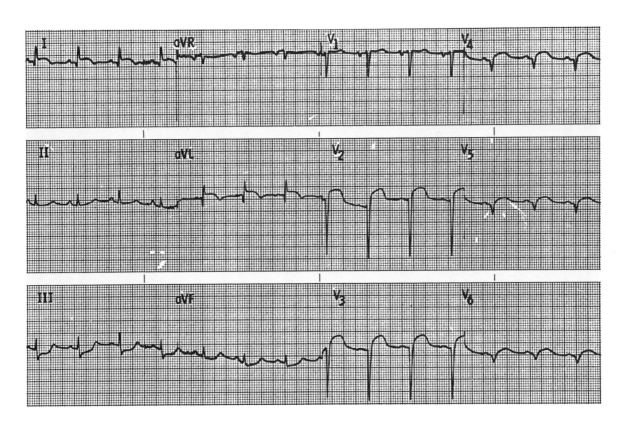

CASE 53: DIAGNOSIS

The cardiac rhythm is sinus with a rate of 85 beats per minute. The diagnosis of extensive anterior myocardial infarction can be entertained without any difficulty because of Q-S waves in leads V_3 through V_6 with embryonic R waves in leads V_1 and V_2 associated with marked elevation of the S-T segment.

However, the persisting and marked S-T segment elevation lasting more than 1 week is extremely unusual for uncomplicated recent myocardial infarction. This patient was found to have a huge ventricular aneurysm, and he eventually expired from intractable congestive heart failure.

The S-T segment depression in leads III and aVF represents a reciprocal change. It can be readily recognized that the abnormal Q waves with S-T segment elevation and T wave inversion are present in leads I and aVL because of the high lateral wall involvement.

chapter 4

MYOCARDITIS AND PERICARDITIS

CASE 54

A 23-year-old woman was admitted to the Intermediate Coronary Care Unit because of a sharp pleuritic chest pain of acute onset.

What is your ECG diagnosis?

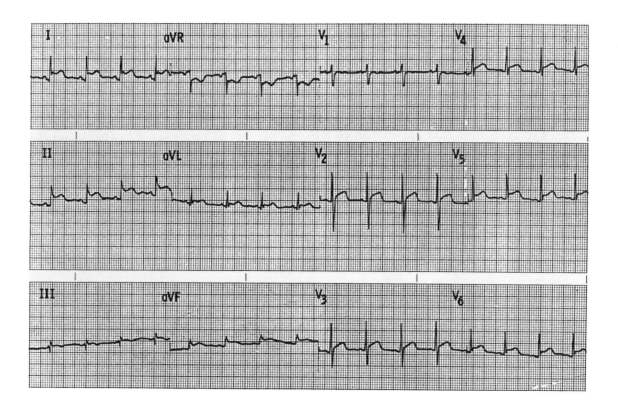

CASE 54: DIAGNOSIS

Cardiac rhythm is normal sinus rhythm with a rate of 100 beats per minute.

It is obvious that S-T segment elevation is present practically in all leads except for leads aVR and V_1. This ECG finding is an early phase of acute pericarditis. It should be noted that there is no pathologic Q wave in any lead.

Since pericarditis is diffuse in nature regardless of its etiology, the electrocardiographic abnormalities usually involve many leads. During the early phase of acute pericarditis, upward elevation of the concave S-T segment occurs diffusely in practically all leads except for lead aVR (sometimes lead V_1 as well). Because of the diffuse process in pericarditis, no reciprocal depression of the S-T segment is observed. It should be remembered that acute myocardial infarction characteristically produces a reciprocal S-T segment depression in the leads facing the uninvolved myocardium during the first 72 hours (see Cases 35, 44, and 46).

During the late stage (*e.g.,* subacute and chronic phases) of pericarditis, the S-T segment elevation returns to the isoelectric line, and the T waves begin to be involved. The T wave inversion in pericarditis may last for weeks or months (see Cases 58, 59, and 60-B). Low voltage of the QRS complexes is very common in chronic pericarditis, particularly in constrictive pericarditis and in massive pericardial effusion (see Cases 69 and 70). In some cases with pericardial effusion, the QRS amplitude becomes so low that the ECG tracing appears to be the isoelectric line in many leads (see Case 70). Abnormal Q waves never occur in uncomplicated pericarditis.

This patient was found to have idiopathic pericarditis.

CASE 55

A 26-year-old woman was admitted to the Coronary Care Unit because of severe chest pain associated with cough and high fever of 24 hours' duration. This illness was preceded by a vague "cold-like" syndrome for 4–5 days. She was extremely sick on admission, and she expired within 48 hours after admission.

What is your ECG diagnosis?

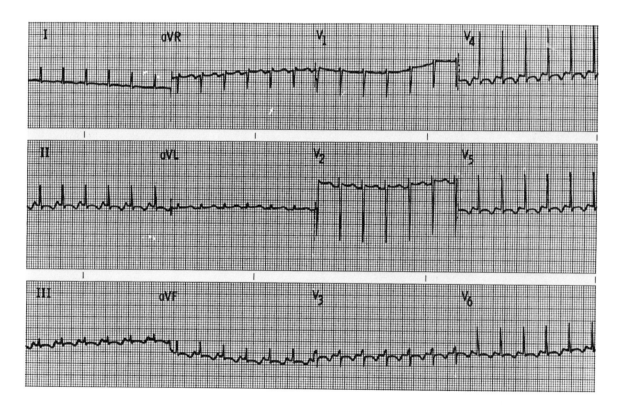

CASE 55: DIAGNOSIS

The cardiac rhythm is marked sinus tachycardia with a rate of 150 beats per minute.

There are inverted T waves involving many leads, and this ECG finding is compatible with sub-acute pericarditis. The S-T segment elevation is no longer present. The electrocardiographic abnormalities due to pericarditis are described in detail elsewhere (see Case 54).

Postmortem examination disclosed evidence of viral pericarditis. No other disease process that could be responsible for her death following a relatively short illness was demonstrated at autopsy in this patient.

CASE 56

An emotionally disturbed 23-year-old man was brought to the emergency room because of a gunshot wound in the chest. He was admitted to the Surgical Cardiac Care Unit immediately for further evaluation and management.

What is your ECG diagnosis?

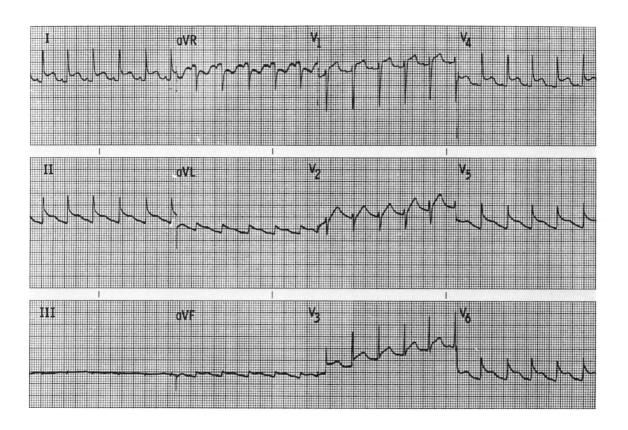

CASE 56: DIAGNOSIS

Cardiac rhythm is marked sinus tachycardia with a rate of 138 beats per minute.

The striking ECG abnormality is marked S-T segment elevation in practically all leads as a result of acute pericarditis. In the early stage of acute pericarditis, the T waves are usually upright.

This patient was found to have purulent bacterial pericarditis which required massive antibiotic therapy.

He recovered completely from acute pericarditis that was a result of a gunshot wound. Psychiatric consultation was requested for his disturbed mental status.

CASE 57

An 8-year-old girl was admitted to the Pediatric Cardiology Service via the emergency room because she was found to have heart murmur associated with fever and arthralgia.

    1. What is your ECG diagnosis?
    2. What is the most likely underlying disorder responsible for the ECG change?

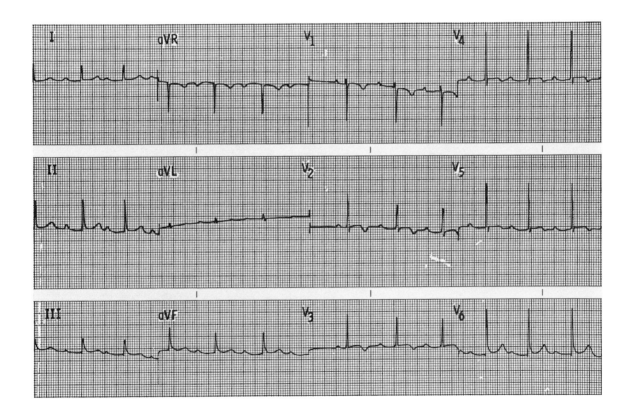

CASE 57: DIAGNOSIS

It is readily recognized that the P-R interval is markedly prolonged in most areas (P-R interval 0.30–0.32 second). In addition, the P-R intervals vary slightly from time to time. Furthermore, the sixth P wave is not followed by the QRS complex and the P-R interval following a ventricular pause is markedly shortened (the seventh QRS complex). Thus, this ECG tracing shows first degree A-V block with an area of Wenckebach A-V block (a transition between the unipolar leads and leads V_1 through V_3).

It has been shown that first degree A-V block is the earliest and the most common ECG finding in acute rheumatic fever. In addition, Wenckebach A-V block is not uncommon in acute rheumatic fever when the A-V conduction is further delayed.

Another ECG finding is the juvenile T wave pattern (inverted T waves in leads V_1 through V_3) which is a normal finding in children and young adults.

She was found to have acute rheumatic fever.

CASE 58

This electrocardiogram was obtained from a 16-month-old boy with high fever. Several days prior to admission, this boy had developed a "cold-like syndrome."

What is your ECG diagnosis?

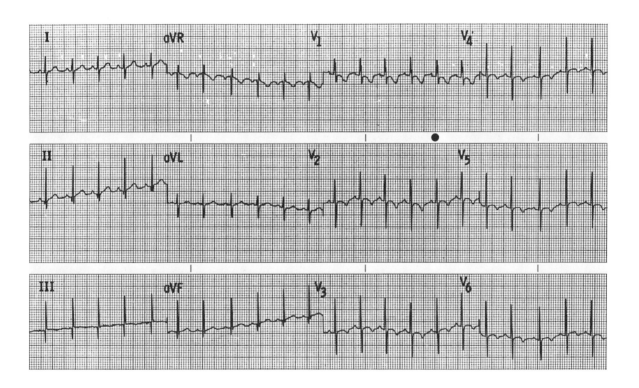

CASE 58: DIAGNOSIS

The cardiac rhythm is sinus tachycardia with a rate of 132 beats per minute.

It should be noted that the T waves are inverted in leads V_1 through V_6, and this ECG finding is compatible with acute myocarditis. The R wave in lead V_1 is relatively tall, and the QRS axis is about $+90°$. These findings are considered to be normal variants for this age group.

The most common ECG finding in acute myocarditis is diffuse T wave changes, particularly inverted T waves involving practically every lead. Other electrocardiographic abnormalities may include A-V block, left or right bundle branch block, diffuse intraventricular block, and extrasystoles of various origins. First degree A-V block is one of the most reliable signs of diagnosing rheumatic carditis in children (see Case 57).

It should be stressed, however, that myocarditis and pericarditis often coexist. It is difficult or often impossible to distinguish between the ECG findings in myocarditis and those of subacute or chronic pericarditis (see Case 54).

This child was found to have viral myocarditis.

CASE 59

This ECG tracing was obtained from a 59-year-old man who has been taking procaine amide (Pronestyl) (500 mg) every 6 hours for 6 months because of frequent ventricular premature contractions. He was admitted to the hospital because he was found to have lupus erythematosus-like syndrome.

What is your ECG diagnosis?

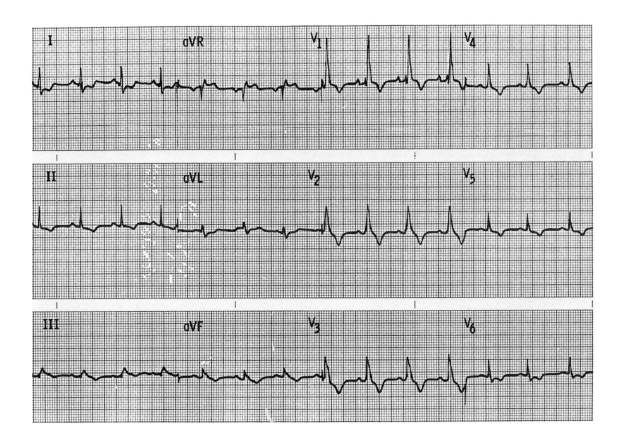

CASE 59: DIAGNOSIS

The cardiac rhythm is sinus with a rate of 90 beats per minute.

The diagnosis of right bundle branch block can be made readily on the basis of RR′ complex in lead V_1 with slurred S waves in leads I, aVL, and V_6 (see Chapter 10).

However, the T wave inversion involving all precordial leads and many limb leads is *not* due to right bundle branch block. That is, this T wave change represents pericarditis as a result of Pronestyl-induced lupus erythematosus-like syndrome.

It has been well documented that some patients may develop lupus erythematosus-like syndrome when receiving procaine amide for 6 months or more. In addition to procaine amide, hydralazine (Apresoline), diphenylhydantoin (Dilantin), and methyldopa (Aldomet) may induce antinuclear antibodies. Some individuals may develop full-blown pictures of lupus erythematosus-like syndrome induced by these agents.

It must be noted that right bundle block in this ECG tracing is the pre-existing abnormality.

CASE 60

An 81-year-old man who had suffered from "heart attack" 6 weeks previously, was re-admitted to the Coronary Care Unit because of recurrent sharp chest pain. The chest pain was said to be aggravated by deep inspiration, particularly with the patient in the supine position. The ECG shown in this page was obtained on admission (tracing A), while another ECG shown on the next page was obtained 1 week later (tracing B).

What is your ECG diagnosis?

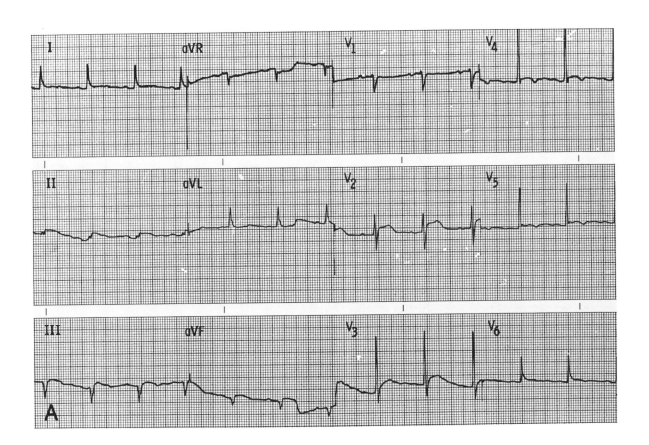

CASE 60: DIAGNOSIS

In tracing *A*, the cardiac rhythm is sinus with a rate of 77 beats per minute. There is an evidence of diaphragmatic (inferior) myocardial infarction which had occurred 6 weeks prior to the present admission, but the S-T segment is elevated diffusely in many leads, associated with slight T wave inversion in some leads. These ECG findings are indicative of pericarditis.

In tracing *B*, the rhythm is again sinus with a rate of 84 beats per minute. Now, the S-T segment elevation is no longer present, but the T wave inversion is much more pronounced. The evidence of old diaphragmatic myocardial infarction is again seen.

Pleuropericarditis secondary to myocardial infarction, generally occuring 2–11 weeks after the acute episode is termed the post-myocardial infarction syndrome (Dressler's syndrome).

An autoimmune etiology is suspected because of the frequent demonstration of anti-myocardial antibodies in the patients, in addition to a favorable response to steroids.

The patient may experience a recurrence of chest pain weeks to months after the acute episode of myocardial infarction. The chest discomfort is sharp in character, and it is usually precordial but may radiate to the shoulder or into the neck. The chest pain is aggravated by deep respiratory movements and by recumbency in many cases.

A pericardial friction rub is the most important physical diagnostic feature. There may be associated low-grade fever, tachycardia, and evidence of pleural or pericardial effusion, and rales may be heard in the chest.

There are no specific laboratory findings. Radiologic studies may reveal pulmonary infiltrates or pleural effusion, but a globular-shaped heart may be seen only if there is a large pericardial effusion. The electrocardiogram classically demonstrates diffuse S-T segment elevation without reciprocal changes in addition to pre-existing myocardial infarction (see tracing *A*). Diagnosis is made on the basis of recurrent chest pain after an appropriate interval following acute myocardial infarction and physical findings as described as above.

Hemorrhagic pericardial effusions and pericardial tamponade are known complications, particularly if anticoagulants are administered in the presence of pericarditis.

Relief of pain may be achieved with aspirin in some instances although protracted or severe discomfort may call for the use of corticosteroids. Prednisone may be started at a dose of 40–60 mg daily, often resulting in dramatic relief of symptoms. The dose is slowly decreased over a 4-week period. Symptoms will often recur when lower dosage levels have been reached or the drug has been withdrawn, necessitating reinstitution of steroids, sometimes for prolonged periods of time.

Prognosis is good in most cases, and the post-myocardial infarction syndrome has not been shown to alter the prognosis of the underlying coronary heart disease.

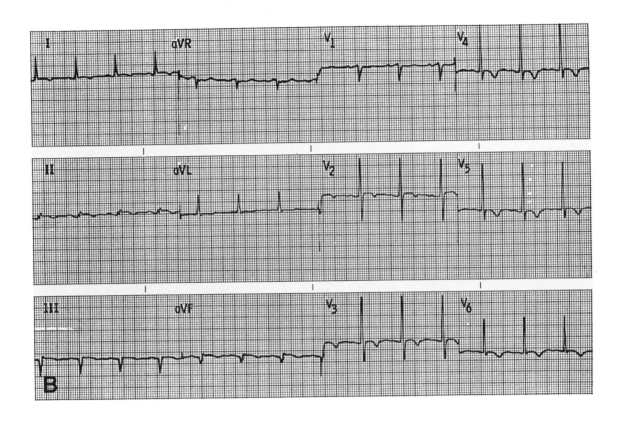

CASE 61

This electrocardiogram was obtained from a 17-year-old girl approximately 2 weeks after surgical repair of a congenital heart disease.

1. *What is your ECG diagnosis?*
2. *What is the most likely underlying cardiac lesion?*

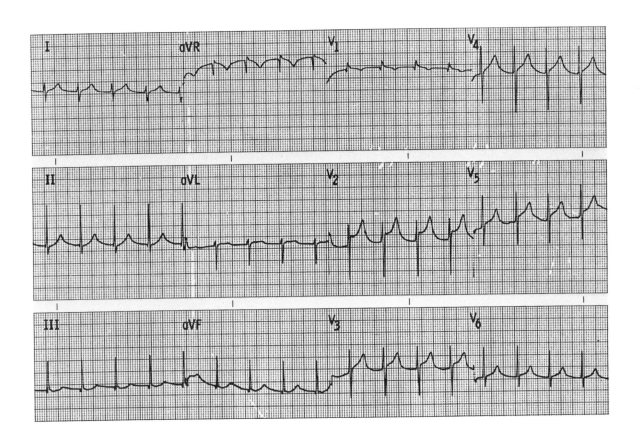

CASE 61: DIAGNOSIS

No P wave is discernible in this ECG tracing, but the ventricular cycles are regular throughout. Thus, the cardiac rhythm is nonparoxysmal A-V junctional tachycardia with a rate of 102 beats per minute (see Chapter 7). It has been shown that nonparoxysmal A-V junctional tachycardia is extremely common postoperatively, particularly following cardiac surgery.

The S-T segment is elevated diffusely in many leads and this ECG finding is indicative of acute pericarditis (see Case 54). The term "post-cardiotomy syndrome" has been used to designate the pericarditis due to cardiac trauma including various surgical procedures.

The underlying cardiac lesion is atrial septal defect, ostium secundum type in which bundle branch block *pattern* is nearly always (up to 90–95% of cases) present (see Case 27).

The post-cardiotomy syndrome is a febrile illness with pericardial and sometimes pleuropulmonary reaction that follows pericardiotomy by 2 weeks to 3 months. It occurs after approximately 30% of pericardiotomies.

Post-cardiotomy syndrome may be due to various causes including cardiac surgery, penetrating trauma to the chest, blunt trauma to the chest, and artificial pacemaker implantation.

The exact pathophysiology of this syndrome remains controversial. Prominent theories include infectious agents, hypersensitivity to blood in the pericardium, and autoimmunity to damaged myocardial or pericardial tissue.

As in other forms of pericarditis, there is chest pain which is intensified by inspiration and recumbency. There may be cough and dyspnea. Unexplained prolongation of postoperative fever or reappearance of fever weeks after surgery are typical. Pericardial and/or pleural effusions may be present and a pericardial friction rub is commonly heard.

Radiologic and electrocardiographic findings, if present, are identical to those described in Dressler's syndrome except for the absence of myocardial infarction pattern (see Case 60).

Corticosteroid therapy induces prompt defervescence and alleviation of symptoms, although relapses are common when therapy is withdrawn. Salicylates may be helpful when symptoms are less severe. Prognosis is good in most cases.

CASE 62

This ECG tracing was obtained from a 19-year-old boy with aortic stenosis 3 weeks after aortic valve replacement.

What is your ECG diagnosis?

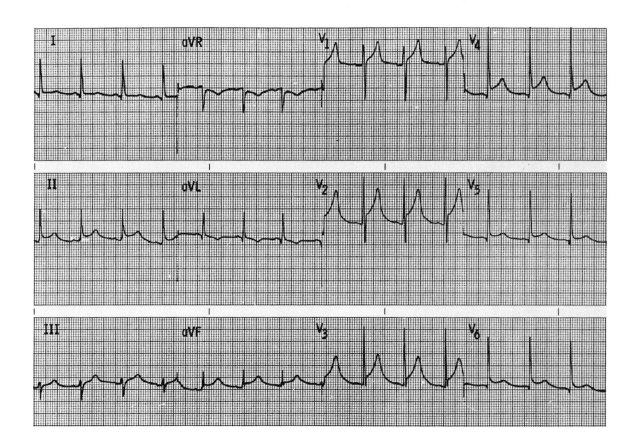

CASE 62: DIAGNOSIS

The cardiac rhythm is sinus with a rate of 85 beats per minute.

It is easy to appreciate the S-T segment elevation diffusely involving many leads. This ECG finding is a typical example of acute pericarditis—the post-cardiotomy syndrome. Detailed descriptions of the post-cardiotomy syndrome are found elsewhere (see Case 61).

In addition, left ventricular hypertrophy is suggested on the basis of the voltage criteria (see Case 10).

CASE 63

This electrocardiogram was obtained from an 11-year-old boy approximately 6 weeks after surgical repair of atrial septal defect, ostium secundum type.

What is your ECG diagnosis?

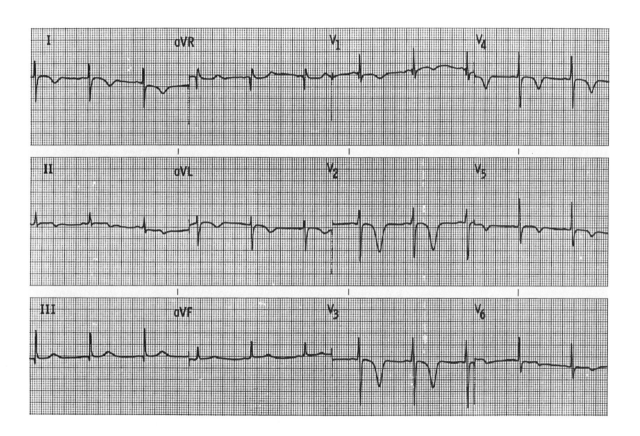

CASE 63: DIAGNOSIS

Cardiac rhythm is sinus with a rate of 63 beats per minute.

There are inverted T waves in practically all leads. This ECG abnormality represents subacute or chronic pericarditis (see Case 54). This is another example of post-cardiotomy syndrome in which the acute phase of pericarditis is over. The T wave inversion in the post-cardiotomy syndrome may last weeks or even months as a manifestation of chronic pericarditis even if the patient is asymptomatic.

The usual ECG abnormalities characteristic of atrial septal defect, ostium primum defect, consist of incomplete right bundle branch block *pattern* with right axis deviation (QRS axis +105°) indicative of right ventricular hypertrophy.

CASE 64

The ECG tracing shown on this page (tracing A) was obtained from an 11-year-old girl with a congenital heart disease, 2 weeks after cardiac surgery. Another ECG shown on the next page (tracing B) was taken 3–4 days later.

1. *What is your ECG diagnosis?*
2. *What is the underlying cardiac lesion?*

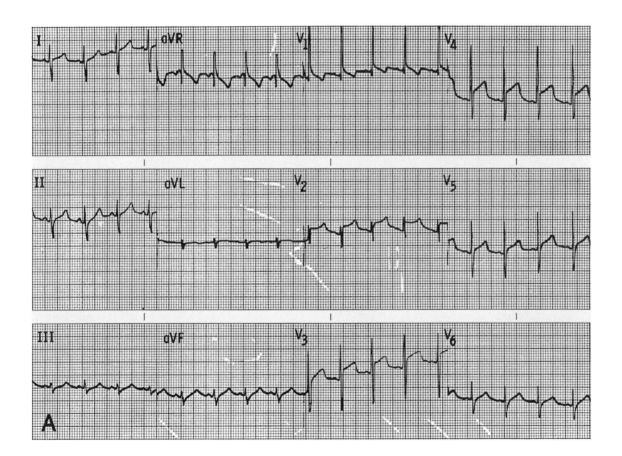

CASE 64: DIAGNOSIS

In tracing A, the cardiac rhythm is sinus tachycardia with a rate of 115 beats per minute. It should be noted that the S-T segment is elevated diffusely, particularly in leads V_2 through V_5. This ECG finding represents acute pericarditis—the post-cardiotomy syndrome. Right ventricular hypertrophy is diagnosed on the basis of a tall R wave in lead V_1 with marked right axis deviation (QRS axis $+210°$). When dealing with the ECG findings shown in this case, the underlying lesion is usually congenital pulmonic stenosis.

The S-T segment elevation is no longer present in the ECG tracing taken 3–4 days later (tracing B).

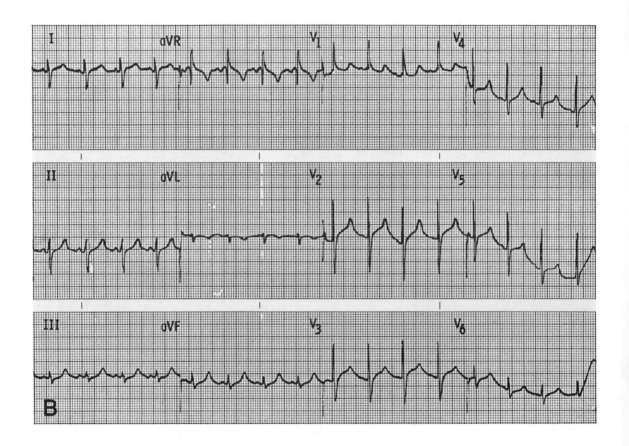

CASE 65

A 65-year-old woman underwent aortocoronary bypass surgery. She had suffered from "heart attack" 3 months previously.

What is your ECG diagnosis?

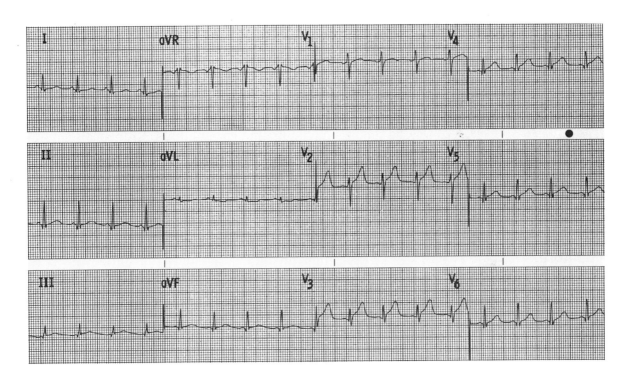

CASE 65: DIAGNOSIS

The cardiac rhythm is sinus tachycardia with a rate of 102 beats per minute. The P-R interval is short (P-R interval 0.08 second), and as indicated previously (see Case 7), the short P-R interval is relatively common during any stressful situation, such as a postoperative period.

It should be noted that the S-T segment is diffusely elevated in many leads because of acute pericarditis—post-cardiotomy syndrome (see Case 61).

The evidence of diaphragmatic-posterolateral myocardial infarction is present in this tracing, and she had suffered from myocardial infarction 3 months previously.

CASE 66

This ECG tracing was obtained from a 38-year-old man 4 weeks after aortocoronary bypass surgery. He had suffered from "heart attack" 6 months previously.

What is your ECG diagnosis?

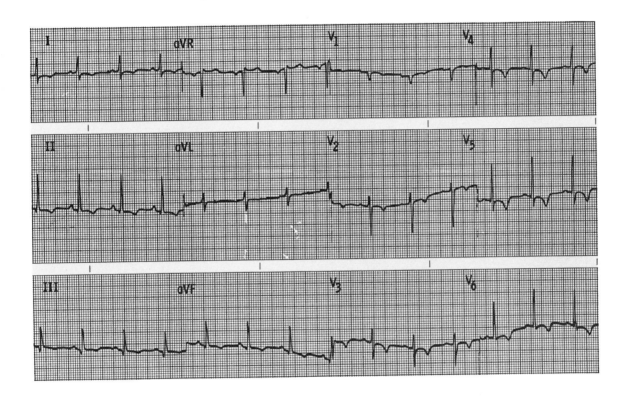

CASE 66: DIAGNOSIS

The cardiac rhythm is sinus with a rate of 83 beats per minute.

   In addition to the evidence of old diaphragmatic (inferior) myocardial infarction, there is T wave inversion diffusely involving practically all leads. This T wave abnormality represents subacute or chronic stage of pericarditis—the post-cardiotomy syndrome. The S-T segment elevation is no longer present in this tracing. The detailed descriptions of pericarditis and post-cardiotomy syndrome are found elsewhere (see Cases 54 and 61).

CASE 67

A 25-year-old black woman with a known sarcoidosis was admitted to the hospital because of congestive heart failure.

What is your ECG diagnosis?

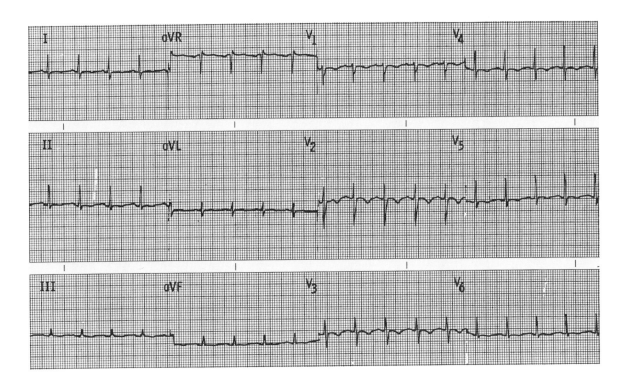

CASE 67: DIAGNOSIS

The cardiac rhythm is sinus tachycardia with a rate of 115 beats per minute. It is noteworthy that the T wave inversion is present diffusely in practically all leads. This ECG finding most likely represents myocardial involvement as a manifestation of multiple organs involvement by sarcoidosis. In a broad term, it is a form of cardiomyopathy.

In addition to diffuse S-T, T wave changes, the patient with sarcoidosis may develop A-V block of various degrees, bundle branch block, and diffuse intraventricular block when the heart is involved directly by the disease. When the patient develops chronic cor-pulmonale secondary to pulmonary sarcoidosis, there may be other ECG abnormalities including right ventricular hypertrophy, right atrial hypertrophy (P-pulmonale), and various atrial tachyarrhythmias.

CASE 68

A 21-year-old black woman was admitted to the hospital because of sickle cell crisis. The patient developed congestive heart failure.

What is your ECG diagnosis?

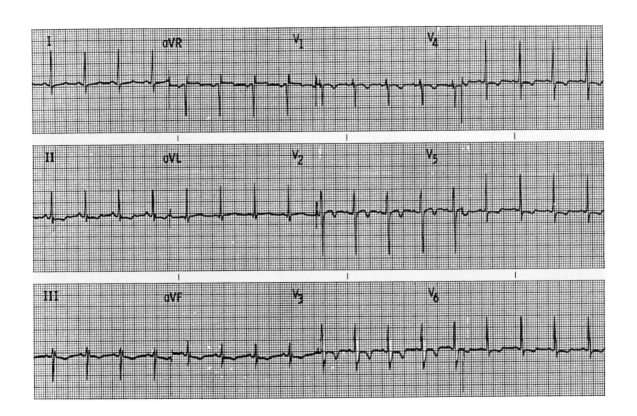

CASE 68: DIAGNOSIS

The cardiac rhythm is sinus with a rate of 100 beats per minute.

The juvenile T wave pattern (see Case 2) can be considered because of the inverted T waves in the precordial leads. However, it is unlikely that the diffuse T wave change involving practically all leads represents the juvenile T wave pattern alone.

The diffuse S-T, T wave change as seen in this ECG tracing is not uncommon when the patient with sickle cell anemia develops congestive heart failure. Significant cardiac damage should be considered in this case. The incidence of congestive heart failure and ECG abnormalities increases progressively as the patient with sickle cell anemia gets older.

CASE 69

This electrocardiogram was obtained from an 18-year-old man with a massive pericardial effusion due to malignancy.

What is your ECG diagnosis?

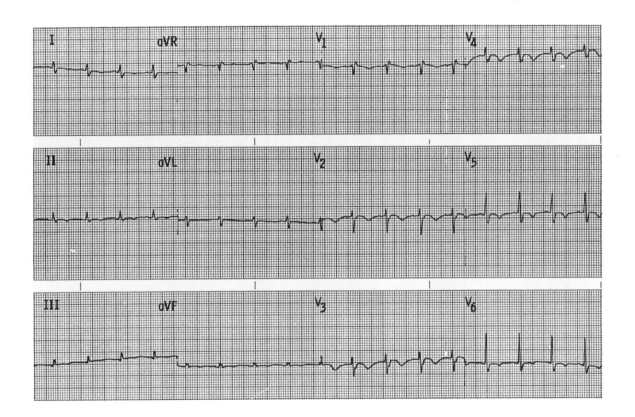

CASE 69: DIAGNOSIS

The cardiac rhythm is sinus tachycardia with a rate of 105 beats per minute.

It is obvious that the T waves are inverted diffusely, involving practically all leads. This ECG finding represents subacute or chronic pericarditis (see Case 54). The S-T segment is not elevated because the acute phase of pericarditis is over.

The amplitude of the QRS complexes is markedly diminished, particularly in the extremity leads. As previously described (see Case 32), the low voltage of the QRS complexes is a rule rather than exception in patients with a massive pericardial effusion.

CASE 70

This electrocardiogram was obtained from an 80-year-old man with a long-standing rheumatoid disease. He has been taking digoxin (0.25 mg) daily for 5 days a week for chronic congestive heart failure associated with atrial fibrillation.

What is your ECG diagnosis?

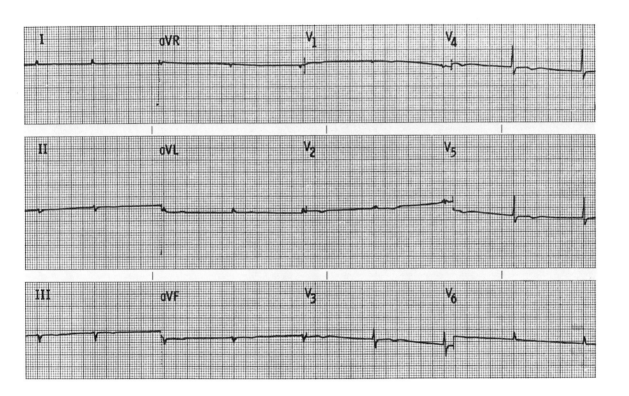

CASE 70: DIAGNOSIS

The atrial activity is not discernible, but the ventricular cycles are regular throughout except for the first R-R interval of the tracing. The cardiac rhythm of this patient is atrial fibrillation with advanced A-V block (see Chapter 8) producing A-V junctional escape rhythm (rate 50 beats per minute). Note a ventricular captured beat (normally a conducted atrial fibrillation beat) in the limb leads (the second QRS complex).

Markedly low voltage of the QRS complexes is evident as a result of rheumatoid pericardial effusion. There are diffuse S-T, T wave changes which are considered to be due to pericarditis and/or digitalis effect.

Atrioventricular junctional escape rhythm due to advanced A-V block is considered to be a manifestation of digitalis toxicity although A-V block induced by rheumatoid disease cannot be excluded entirely.

chapter 5

DISTURBANCES OF SINUS IMPULSE FORMATION AND CONDUCTION

CASE 71

This electrocardiogram was obtained from a 69-year-old man with bronchogenic carcinoma.

What is your ECG diagnosis?

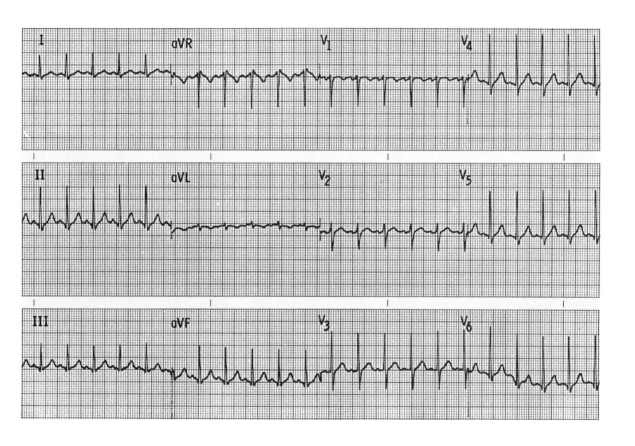

CASE 71: DIAGNOSIS

Cardiac rhythm is sinus tachycardia with a rate of 134 beats per minute. This ECG tracing is otherwise within normal limits.

The diagnostic criteria of sinus tachycardia are the same as those of normal sinus rhythm (see Case 1), except that the sinus rate is faster than 100 beats per minute.

Thus, the diagnostic criteria of sinus tachycardia include:

1. P waves of sinus origin (P axis 0 to +90°).
2. Constant P wave configuration in a given lead.
3. Constant and normal P-R interval (between 0.12 and 0.20 second).
4. Sinus rate between 101–160 beats per minute (faster than 160 and up to 200 during physical exercise).
5. Regular P-P cycles.

Sinus tachycardia is extremely common during any stressful situation, particularly in those patients with malignancy.

CASE 72

A 34-year-old man with congestive heart failure due to idiopathic cardiomyopathy was admitted to the Cardiology Service.

What is your cardiac rhythm diagnosis?

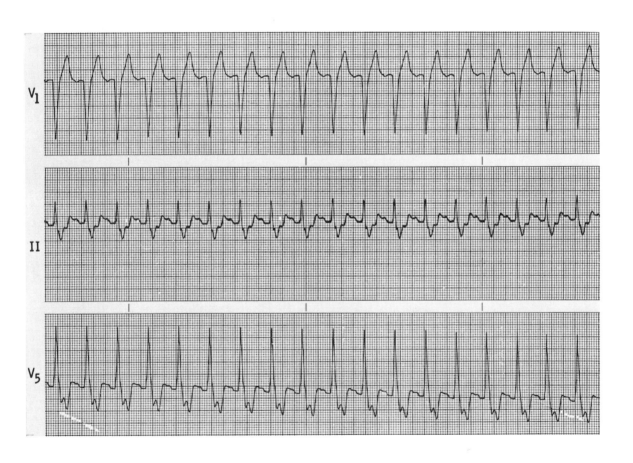

CASE 72: DIAGNOSIS

The cardiac rhythm is sinus tachycardia with a rate of 116 beats per minute.

It is obvious that the QRS complexes are broad and bizarre. This ECG abnormality is diffuse or nonspecific intraventricular block which is *not* due to right or left bundle branch block (see Chapter 10). Ectopic tachycardia, particularly nonparoxysmal ventricular tachycardia (idioventricular tachycardia or accelerated ventricular rhythm; see Chapter 9) is closely simulated.

It has been shown that nonspecific (diffuse) intraventricular block is common in patients with idiopathic cardiomyopathy.

CASE 73

This electrocardiogram was obtained from a 17-year-old girl during her annual checkup.

What is your cardiac rhythm diagnosis?

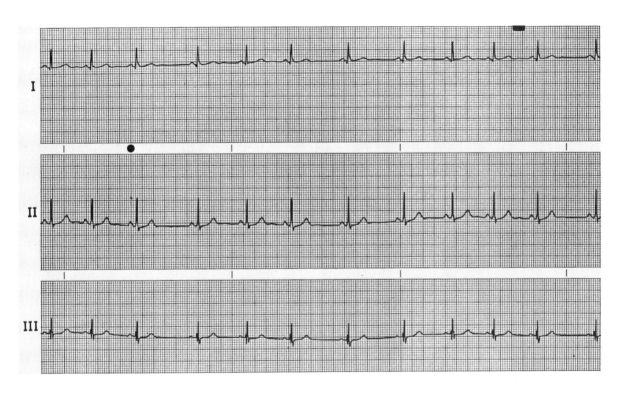

CASE 73: DIAGNOSIS

Cardiac rhythm is sinus arrhythmia with a rate ranging from 62–78 beats. Sinus arrthythmia is a rule rather than an exception in children and young adults.

Sinus arrhythmia is diagnosed when the P-P cycles in sinus rhythm vary 0.16 second or more. Sinus arrhythmia is frequently associated with sinus bradycardia, particularly in children and young adults, and is occasionally associated with sinus tachycardia. The presence of sinus brady-cardia or tachycardia does not preclude the diagnosis of sinus arrhythmia. The diagnostic criteria for sinus arrhythmia are as follows:

1. P wave of sinus origin (P axis between 0 and $+90°$).
2. Constant and normal P-R interval (0.12–0.20 second).
3. Constant P wave configuration in each given lead.
4. Rate between 45–100 beats per minute (occasionally slower than 45 and faster than 100 beats per minute).
5. Irregular P-P cycle (variation of P-P interval 0.16 second or more).

Generally sinus arrhythmia is divided into two major types: respiratory and nonrespiratory. In respiratory sinus arrhythmia, which is most common in healthy young adults, the sinus rate increases gradually with inspiration and slows with expiration as shown in this case. On the other hand, nonrespiratory sinus arrhythmia has no relation to the respiratory cycle. Nonrespiratory sinus arrhythmia is more common in elderly individuals with diseased hearts.

Sinus arrhythmia not uncommonly coexists with wandering atrial pacemaker (see Case 74).

CASE 74

This ECG tracing was obtained from a 10-year-old girl with congenital pulmonic stenosis.

What is your cardiac rhythm diagnosis?

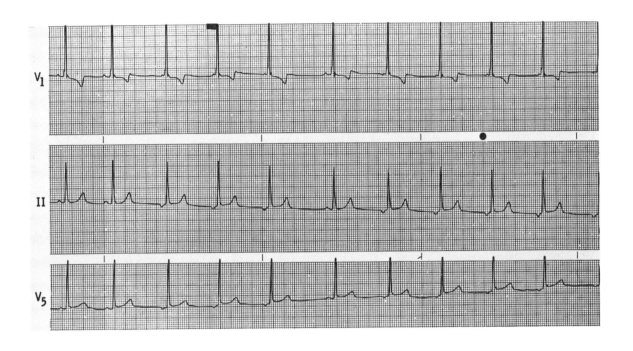

CASE 74: DIAGNOSIS

The cardiac rhythm is sinus arrhythmia with wandering atrial pacemaker (rate 62 beats per minute). Note that P-P cycle is irregular, and the P wave configuration varies.

It has been shown that wandering atrial pacemaker is usually associated with sinus arrhythmia. Hence, many cardiologists consider that wandering atrial pacemaker is an exaggerated form of sinus arrhythmia. For the same reason, wandering atrial pacemaker is clinically insignificant as respiratory sinus arrhythmia.

It is noteworthy that the R wave in lead V_1 is extremely tall because of right ventricular hypertrophy as a result of pulmonic stenosis (see Case 15).

CASE 75

This electrocardiogram was obtained from a 22-year-old athletic man.

What is your cardiac rhythm diagnosis?

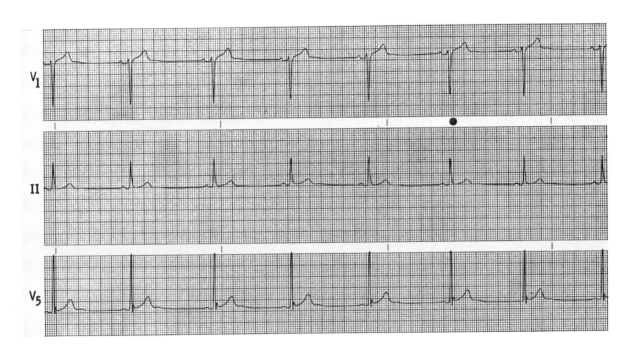

CASE 75: DIAGNOSIS

Cardiac rhythm is marked sinus bradycardia with a rate of 42 beats per minute.

Sinus rhythm with a rate slower than 60 beats per minute is termed sinus bradycardia. The usual rate of sinus bradycardia is between 45–59 beats per minute and occasionally may be as slow as 30–35 beats per minute. Sinus bradycardia is often associated with sinus arrhythmia. However, the presence of sinus arrhythmia does not preclude the diagnosis of sinus bradycardia. The diagnostic criteria of sinus bradycardia include:

1. P wave of sinus origin (P axis 0 to $+90°$).
2. Constant and normal P-R interval (0.12–0.20 second).
3. Constant P wave configuration in each given lead.
4. Rate between 45–59 beats per minute.
5. Regular or slightly irregular P-P cycle.

Sinus bradycardia is common in healthy young adults, particularly in athletes. This finding, of course, is a physiologic phenomenon. On the other hand, sinus bradycardia is commonly induced by various drugs including propranolol (Inderal), digitalis, reserpine (Serpasil), guanethidine (Ismelin), and methyldopa (Aldomet). In addition, sinus bradycardia is common in patients with acute diaphragmatic myocardial infarction. Furthermore, sick sinus syndrome should be suspected when marked bradycardia is found in elderly individuals.

CASE 76

A 78-year-old man with chronic congestive heart failure was admitted to the Intermediate Coronary Care Unit because of digitalis intoxication.

What is your cardiac rhythm diagnosis?

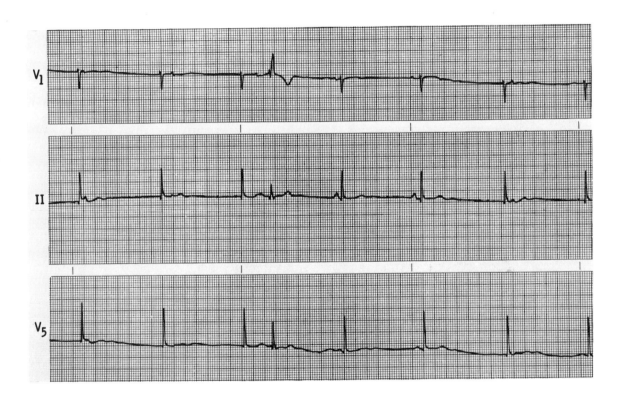

CASE 76: DIAGNOSIS

Arrows indicate sinus P waves. The cardiac rhythm is marked sinus bradycardia (indicated by *arrows;* atrial rate 37 beats per minute) with A-V junctional escape rhythm (rate 43 beats per minute) and occasional ventricular captured beats (normally conducted sinus beats, marked *X*) producing incomplete A-V dissociation (see Chapter 8). Note that the first ventricular captured beat (fourth QRS complex) exhibits aberrant ventricular conduction because of a short coupling interval. The ventricular captured beat with aberrant ventricular conduction closely resembles a ventricular premature contraction.

Whenever the sinus rate becomes the same as or slower than the inherent rate of the subsidiary pacemakers, A-V junction may take over the ventricular activity to produce complete or incomplete A-V dissociation (see Chapter 7).

Marked sinus bradycardia with or without A-V junctional escape rhythm is one of the most common digitalis-induced arrhythmias. When the ventricular rate is very slow (45 beats or less) or the patient is symptomatic (dizziness, hypotension, fainting, etc.) from the digitalis-induced sinus bradycardia, the use of artificial pacemaker (usually a temporary pacing) should be considered. However, in most cases, discontinuation of digitalis for a few days is sufficient for the treatment of digitalis toxicity.

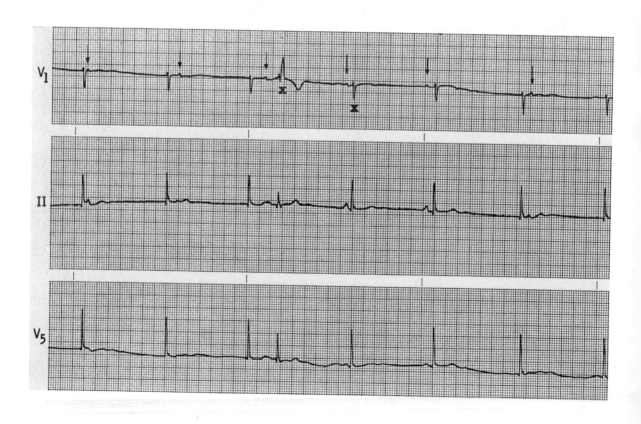

CASE 77

This electrocardiogram was obtained from a 79-year-old man with chronic congestive heart failure. Digitalis toxicity was suspected. There was no history of fainting episodes.

1. What is the cardiac rhythm diagnosis?
2. What is your ECG diagnosis?
3. Is artificial pacing indicated?

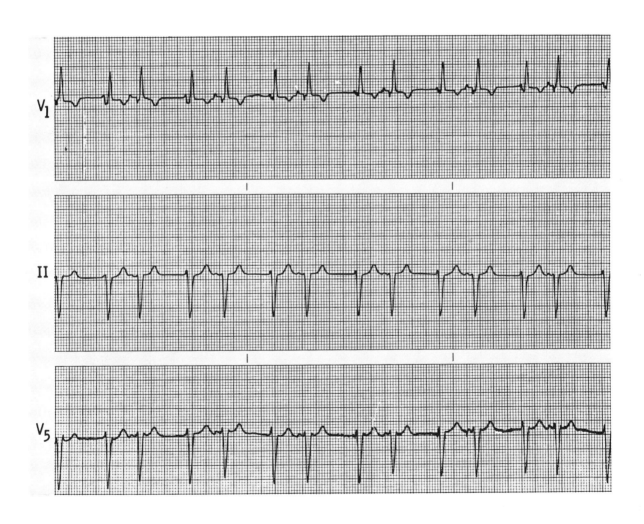

CASE 77: DIAGNOSIS

Arrows indicate sinus P waves. The cardiac rhythm is sinus bradycardia (indicated by *arrows;* atrial rate 48 beats per minute) with A-V junctional escape beats (marked *E*) which occur on every other beat causing a form of bigeminy. This type of bigeminal rhythm has been called "A-V junctional escape-bigeminy." It should be noted that the escape interval (the interval from the QRS complex of the sinus beat to the next A-V junctional escape beat) is shorter than usual A-V junctional escape rhythm. This ECG finding has been termed "accelerated" escape beat or rhythm.

The obvious ECG abnormality in this tracing is a bifascicular block which consists of right bundle branch block and left anterior hemiblock (see Chapter 10).

Artificial pacing is *not* indicated for either asymptomatic bifascicular block or digitalis-induced arrhythmia. It must be remembered that digitalis never produces intraventricular block. In other words, the bifascicular block is the pre-existing ECG abnormality.

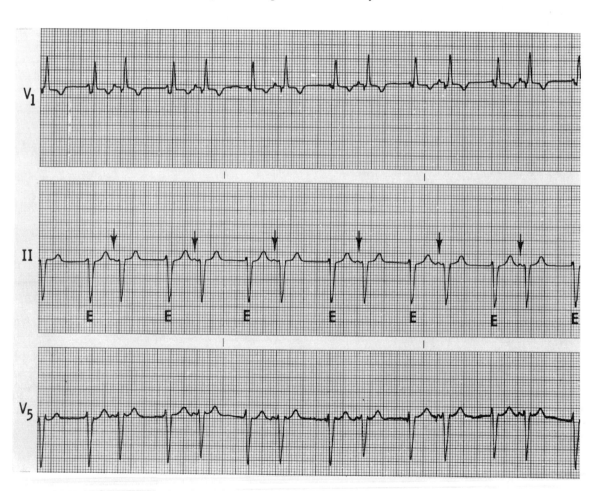

CASE 78

These cardiac rhythm strips were recorded during carotid sinus stimulation from a 70-year-old man with frequent episodes of dizzy spells. He was not taking any drug.

1. *What is your cardiac rhythm diagnosis?*
2. *What is the ECG abnormality?*
3. *What is the treatment of choice?*

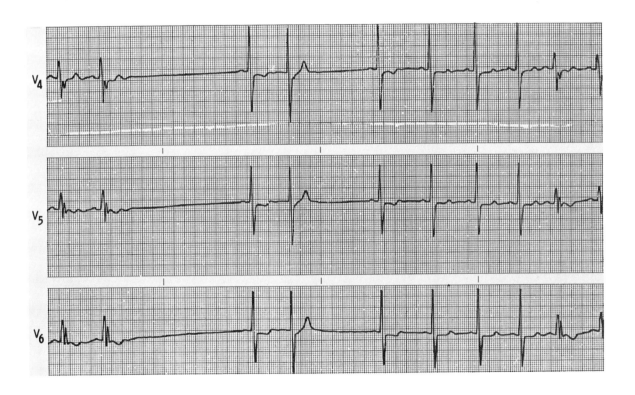

CASE 78: DIAGNOSIS

The cardiac rhythm is sinus arhythmia with areas of sinus arrest induced by carotid sinus stimulation. This phenomenon is called "hypersensitive carotid sinus syndrome." Needless to say, markedly slow heart rate by carotid sinus stimulation is responsible for frequent episodes of dizziness.

An interesting ECG abnormality in this tracing is intermittent left bundle branch block and left anterior hemiblock (see Chapter 10). That is, the left posterior fascicle recovers from its refractoriness when the heart rate slows significantly so that left bundle branch block transforms to left anterior hemiblock during the slower heart rate. The diagnosis of intermittent left anterior hemiblock is confirmed by the ECG finding in the limb leads (see Chapter 10).

For the treatment of hypersensitive carotid sinus syndrome a permanent artificial pacemaker (demand unit) implantation is the treatment of choice.

CASE 79

The Holter monitor electrocardiogram was obtained from a 53-year-old man because of frequent episodes of lightheadedness.

    1. What is your rhythm diagnosis?
    2. What is the treatment of choice?

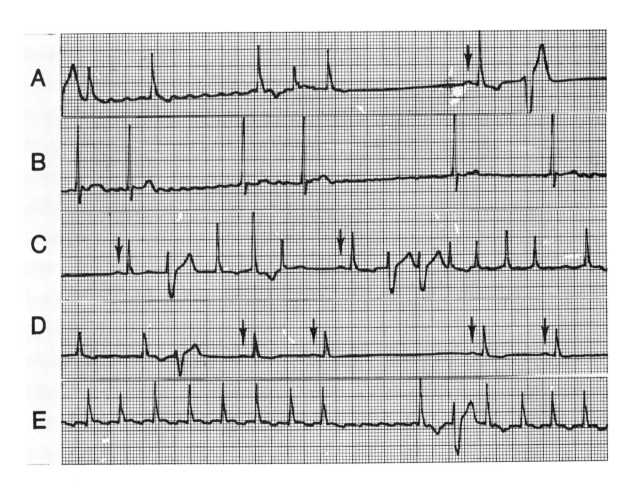

CASE 79: DIAGNOSIS

The rhythm strips *A* to *E* represent lead II, and they are not continuous. *Arrows* indicate sinus P waves. The underlying cardiac rhythm is sinus arrhythmia with areas of sinus arrest. In addition, there are areas of atrial fibrillation with advanced A-V block (strips *A* and *B*), atrial flutter (strip *E*), and frequent ventricular premature contractions (strips *A* and *D*), as well as aberrant ventricular conduction (strips *C* and *E*). These ECG abnormalities represent brady-tachyarrhythmia syndrome as a result of sick sinus syndrome. It should be noted that sick sinus syndrome is the most common underlying disorder responsible for the production of brady-tachyarrhythmia syndrome. Various manifestations of sick sinus syndrome include:

1. Marked sinus bradycardia in elderly individuals.
2. Sinus arrest and sinoatrial block.
3. Chronic atrial fibrillation with advanced A-V block.
4. Chronic atrial fibrillation preceded by or followed by marked sinus bradycardia and/or marked first degree A-V block (P-R interval more than 0.28 second).
5. Prolonged sinus node recovery time by atrial pacing $\geqq$ 1500 msec.
6. Brady-tachyarrhythmia syndrome.
7. Common association with slow A-V junctional escape rhythm, bifascicular or trifascicular block, and complete A-V block.

The treatment of choice for brady-tachyarrhythmia syndrome due to sick sinus syndrome is a permanent artificial pacemaker implantation. In addition to the artificial pacemaker, one or more antiarrhythmic agents may be required if the tachyarrhythmia portion of the sick sinus syndrome is not suppressed by the artificial pacemaker.

CASE 80

These cardiac rhythm strips were obtained from a 68-year-old woman with lightheadedness. She was not taking any drug.

1. What is your cardiac rhythm diagnosis?
2. What is the treatment of choice?

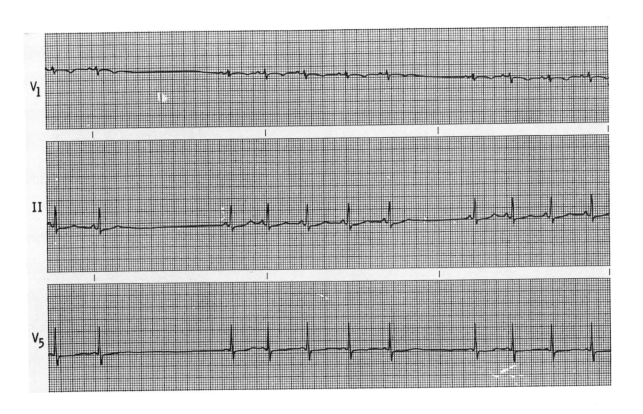

CASE 80: DIAGNOSIS

The underlying cardiac rhythm is sinus arrhythmia with a rate of 85 beats per minute.

The diagnosis of intermittent Mobitz type-II sinoatiral (S-A) block can be made on the basis of the fact that a long P-P interval is a multiple of the basic P-P cycle. Sinotrial block superficially resembles sinus arrest, although the fundamental mechanisms responsible for the production of these rhythm disorders are completely different.

Sinus arrest means that the sinus node is unable to produce a cardiac impulse so that a long pause due to sinus arrest has no relationship to the basic P-P cycle. On the other hand, in S-A block, the sinus node itself produces the impulses as usual, but there is an exit block at the sino-atrial junction. As a result, type-II S-A block produces a long sinus pause which is a multiple of the basic P-P cycle. Type-I (Wenckebach) S-A block is discussed elsewhere (see Case 82).

The underlying process in S-A block is often sick sinus syndrome (see Case 79) for which an artificial pacemaker is indicated if the patient is symptomatic.

CASE 81

A 63-year-old man who had received a permanent artificial pacemaker (fixed-rate unit) implantation 20 months previously was readmitted to the Intermediate Coronary Care Unit because of recurrent fainting episodes.

      1. What is your cardiac rhythm diagnosis?
      2. What is the underlying disorder responsible for this arrhythmia?
      3. What is the status of the artificial pacemaker?

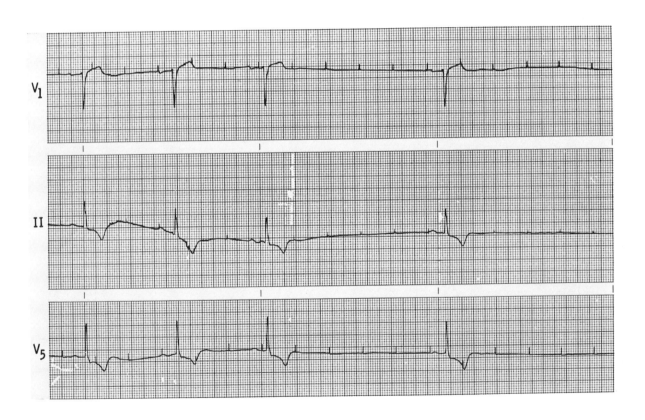

CASE 81: DIAGNOSIS

The underlying cardiac rhythm is marked sinus bradycardia (rate 38 beats per minute) with intermittent Mobitz type-II S-A block (see Case 80) and first degree A-V block (P-R interval 0.26 second). Note that a long P-P interval is twice the length of the basic P-P cycle. As indicated earlier, S-A block is often a manifestation of sick sinus syndrome (see Case 79).

Artificial pacemaker spikes (rate 108 beats per minute) are readily recognized, but none of the pacemaker spikes are followed by QRS complexes. In addition, the pacing rate is markedly enhanced (rate 108 beats per minute) to compare with the pre-set pacing rate of 70 beats per minute. This ECG finding is an obvious example of malfunctioning artificial pacemaker. The accelerated pacing rate due to malfunctioning pacemaker is called "runaway pacemaker."

Note inverted T waves in leads II and V_5 indicative of diaphragmatic-lateral myocardial ischemia.

CASE 82

These cardiac rhythm strips were obtained from a 71-year-old man with possible digitalis toxicity.

What is your cardiac rhythm diagnosis?

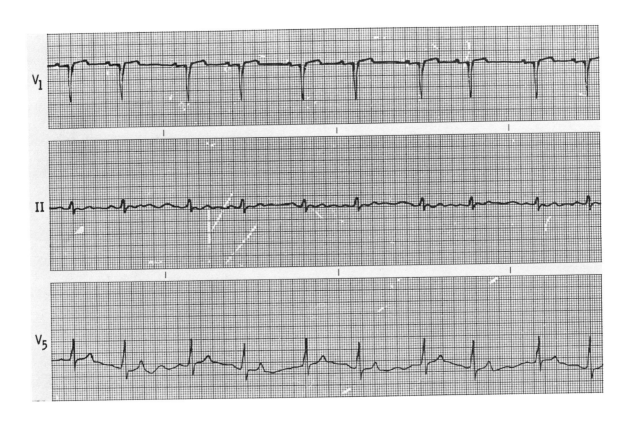

CASE 82: DIAGNOSIS

The basic cardiac rhythm is sinus (rate 90 beats per minute), but the P-P cycles demonstrate a form of bigeminy (pseudo-bigeminy). That is, the short and long P-P cycles alternate throughout the tracing. The long P-P interval is shorter than two short P-P intervals. Yet, the P-R intervals remain constant. This regular irregularity of the P-P cycles represents 3:2 Wenckebach (Mobitz type-I) S-A block. It should be noted that 3:2 Wenckebach S-A block is analogous to 3:2 Wenckebach A-V block except that the level of the block is different.

Wenckebach S-A block is probably the most difficult arrhythmia to understand for most physicians because the direct measurement of the sinus rate is not possible. For better understanding of Wenckebach S-A block, every reader should study Wenckebach A-V block first (see Chapter 8, Cases 131 and 132). Wenckebach A-V block produces a progressive shortening of the R-R cycles whereas Wenckebach S-A block causes a progressive shortening of the P-P cycles until a pause occurs. When the conduction ratio is 3:2, a form of bigeminy (pseudo-bigeminy) is produced so that the short and long cycles alternate.

Note prominent U waves indicative of hypokalemia. Wenckbach S-A block is not too uncommon in digitalis intoxication, and hypokalemia frequently predisposes to digitalis toxicity.

chapter 6

ATRIAL ARRHYTHMIAS

CASE 83

These cardiac rhythm strips were obtained from a 63-year-old woman with slight hypertension. She was not taking any drug.

What is your cardiac rhythm diagnosis?

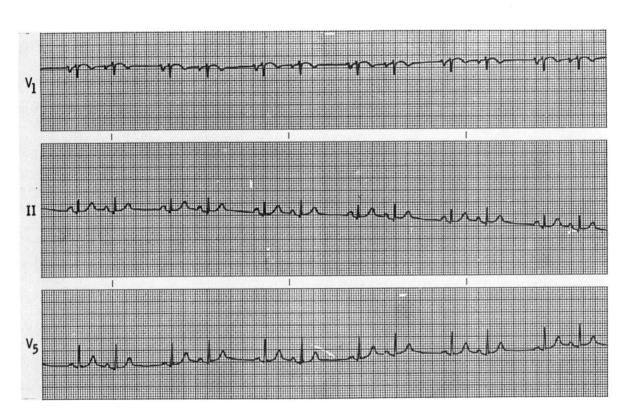

CASE 83: DIAGNOSIS

The basic cardiac rhythm is sinus with a rate of 78 beats per minute. There are frequent atrial premature contractions (indicated by *arrows)* producing atrial bigeminy. It should be noted that the ectopic P waves (indicated by *arrows*) have different configurations as compared to the P waves of sinus origin. When atrial bigeminy is established, the precise measurement of the sinus rate is not possible. This is observed because the sinus node is discharged passively by the atrial premature impulse so that the sinus node loses its automaticity momentarily. This phenomenon is responsible for a pause following each atrial premature contraction. The interval from the ectopic P wave to the following sinus P wave is termed "returning cycle" which is usually longer than the basic sinus P-P cycle because of momentary suppression of the sinus node by the ectopic impulse. Yet, the sinus P-P interval which contains the ectopic P wave is shorter than two basic sinus P-P cycles. As a result, the term "non-full compensatory pause" is used in atrial premature contractions to distinguish it from a full compensatory pause which is observed in ventricular premature contractions in most cases (see Chapter 9).

It can be said that a full compensatory pause is observed as long as the sinus impulse formation is not disturbed. On the other hand, a non-full compensatory pause is produced when the sinus impulse formation is interfered with.

Note evidence of left atrial enlargement (see Case 11).

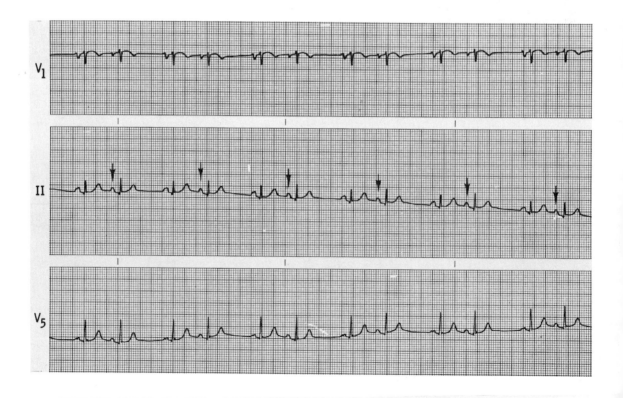

CASE 84

This ECG tracing was obtained from a 59-year-old man with chronic congestive heart failure due to hypertensive heart disease. He has been taking digoxin (0.25 mg) and hydro-chlorothiazide (25 mg) daily.

What is your cardiac rhythm diagnosis?

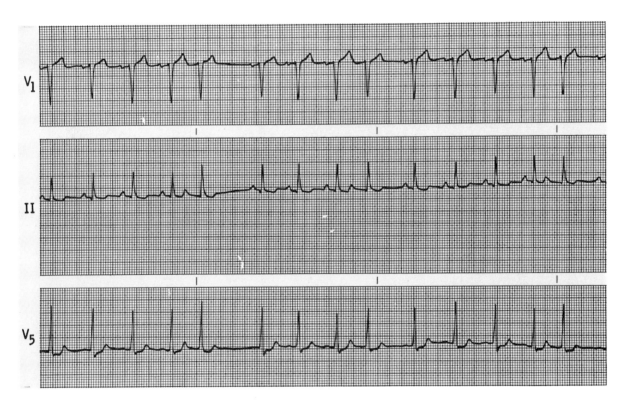

CASE 84: DIAGNOSIS

The underlying cardiac rhythm is sinus with a rate of 93 beats per minute. There are frequent atrial premature contractions (indicated by *arrows*).

It should be noted that the P-R interval of the atrial premature contraction (indicated by *arrows*) is much longer than the P-R interval of the sinus beat. This is due to the fact that the ectopic atrial impulse reaches the A-V junction during a partial refractory period. Thus, atrial premature contractions almost always show longer P-R interval than the sinus beats. When the atrial premature impulse occurs so early that it reaches the A-V junction during an absolute refractory period, needless to say, the atrial impulse will *not* be conducted to the ventricles. This is called "blocked" or "nonconducted" atrial premature contraction (see Case 86). Note slight aberrant ventricular conduction in atrial premature contractions.

Left ventricular hypertrophy is strongly suggested although the left ventricular voltage is not sufficient (see Case 10). In addition, digitalis effect may be responsible for the S-T segment sagging.

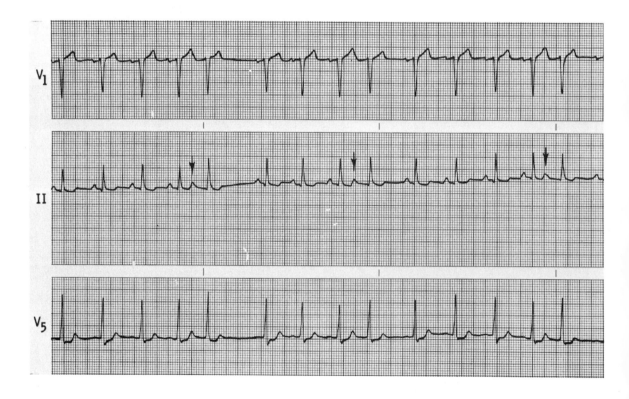

CASE 85

This electrocardiogram was obtained from a 66-year-old woman with mild congestive heart failure due to coronary heart disease. She has been taking digoxin (0.25 mg) daily for several years.

1. *What is your cardiac rhythm diagnosis?*
2. *Is there any evidence of digitalis intoxication electrocardiographically?*

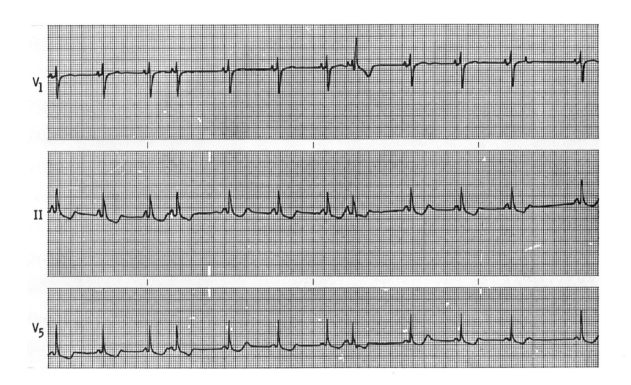

CASE 85: DIAGNOSIS

The underlying cardiac rhythm is sinus with a rate of 68 beats per minute. The P-R interval is relatively short (P-R interval 0.10 second), but there is no definite evidence of Wolff-Parkinson-White syndrome (see Chapter 11). As mentioned previously, the short P-R interval is not uncommon during any stressful situations or among individuals with anxiety.

It should be noted that there are three ectopic P waves (indicated by *arrows*) which closely simulate atrial premature contractions. However, by close observation, one can appreciate the varying coupling intervals (interval from the ectopic beat to the preceding beat of the basic rhythm). In addition, the interectopic intervals (interval between two ectopic beats) are constant. Therefore, the cardiac rhythm diagnosis is atrial parasystole (see also Case 200).

It should be noted that the second parasystolic beat shows aberrant ventricular conduction (marked *X*) because the atrial ectopic impulse is conducted to the ventricles during their partial refractory period. On the other hand, the last atrial parasystolic P wave (marked *O*) is not followed by the QRS complex because the ectopic atrial impulse reaches the ventricles during their absolute refractory period.

Atrial premature contractions and atrial parasystole resemble each other very closely electrocardiographically, but the former may be induced by digitalis while the latter has no relationship to digitalis toxicity.

Diffuse S-T segment sagging represents digitalis effect which has again nothing to do with digitalis toxicity.

The diagnostic criteria of parasystole include:

1. Varying coupling intervals.
2. Constant shortest interectopic intervals.
3. Long interectopic interval shows a multiple of the shortest interectopic interval.
4. Frequent occurrence of fusion beats when a long rhythm strip is available (more common in ventricular parasystole; see Case 200).

Ventricular parasystole is the most common, while A-V junctional or atrial parasystole is only occasionally observed.

It should be reemphasized that ordinary premature beats (particularly those ventricular in origin) are frequently digitalis-induced, whereas parasystole does not seem to have any relationship to digitalis preparation.

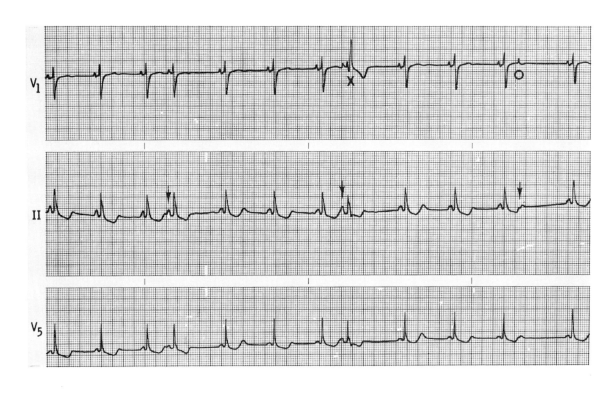

CASE 86

These cardiac rhythm strips were obtained from a 54-year-old woman with systemic lupus erythematosus.

What is your cardiac rhythm diagnosis?

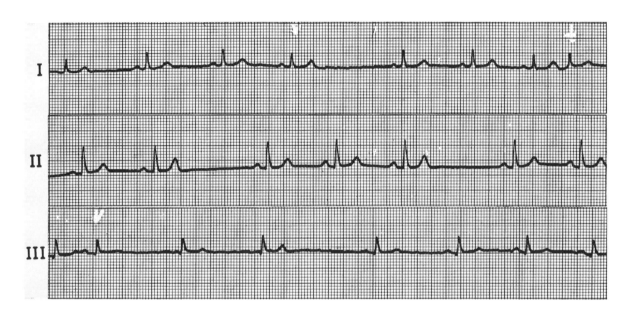

CASE 86: DIAGNOSIS

The underlying cardiac rhythm is sinus arrhythmia with rate ranging from 60–73 beats per minute.

It should be noted that there are frequent atrial premature contractions (indicated by *arrows*), and many of them are not followed by QRS complexes. Thus, the cardiac rhythm diagnosis is frequent nonconducted or blocked atrial premature contractions. Although the coupling intervals vary significantly, atrial parasystole cannot be diagnosed because the parasystolic cycle is not found. That is, the shortest interectopic intervals are not constant (see Case 85).

The cardiac rhythm shown in the tracing superficially appears to be grossly irregular sinus arrhythmia because the majority of the ectopic P waves are superimposed on the tops of the T waves of the preceding beats. Otherwise, nonconducted atrial premature contractions may be erroneously diagnosed as sinus arrest, sinoatrial block (see Chapter 5), or even second degree A-V block (see Chapter 8).

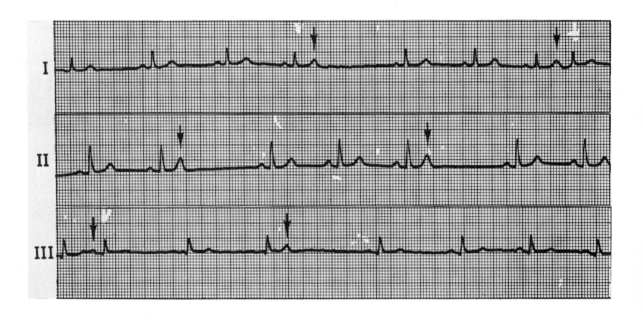

CASE 87

These cardiac rhythm strips were obtained from a 51-year-old woman with coronary heart disease.

What is your cardiac rhythm diagnosis?

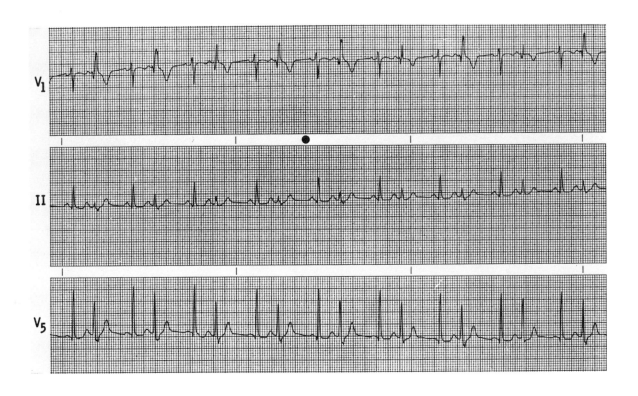

CASE 87: DIAGNOSIS

The underlying cardiac rhythm is sinus tachycardia with a rate of 110 beats per minute.

It is readily recognized that there are frequent ventricular premature contractions (indicated by *arrows*) producing atrial bigeminy. It should be noted that all atrial premature contractions reveal aberrant ventricular conduction, and this finding closely resembles ventricular premature contractions.

In 80–85% of cases, the configuration of aberrant ventricular conduction reveals right bundle branch block pattern. Occasionally, the aberrantly conducted beats may show left anterior hemiblock pattern. Rarely, left bundle branch block pattern (see Case 95) or left posterior hemiblock pattern is observed in aberrant ventricular conduction. At times, aberrant ventricular conduction may exhibit a bifascicular block pattern which consists of right bundle branch block pattern and left anterior or posterior hemiblock pattern (see Case 88).

It is interesting to observe that the degree of aberrant ventricular conduction varies in this ECG tracing. As a result, complete and incomplete right bundle branch block pattern is shown intermittently during aberrant ventricular conduction.

The fundamental reason why aberrant ventricular conduction is extremely common in atrial bigeminy is discussed elsewhere (see Case 88).

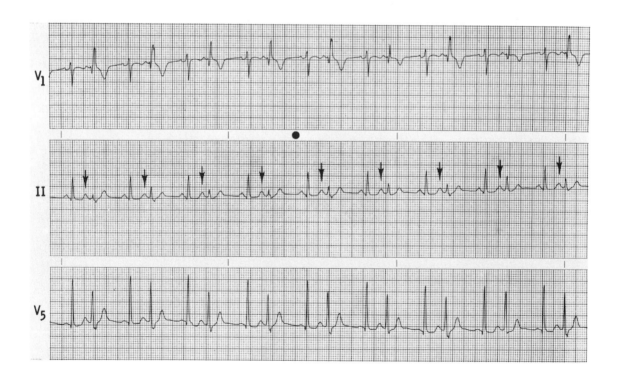

CASE 88

This electrocardiogram was obtained from an 84-year-old man with coronary heart disease.

1. *What is your cardiac rhythm diagnosis?*
2. *What is your ECG diagnosis?*

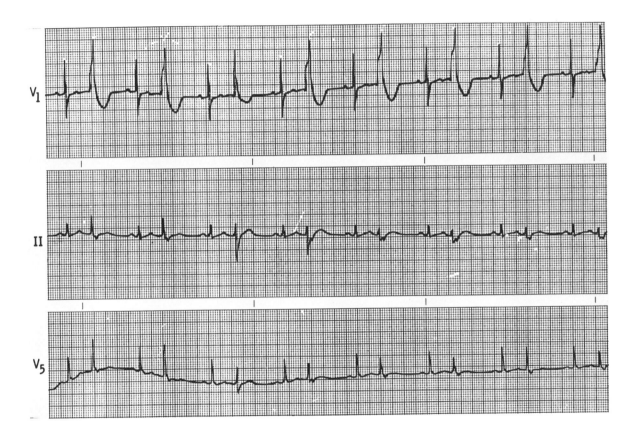

CASE 88: DIAGNOSIS

The underlying cardiac rhythm is sinus with a rate of 100 beats per minute.

There are frequent atrial premature contractions (indicated by *arrows*) producing atrial bigeminy. All atrial premature contractions show bizarre configuration as a result of aberrant ventricular conduction. Again, the ECG finding closely simulates frequent ventricular premature contractions. The aberrantly conducted beats show right bundle branch block pattern with intermittent left anterior hemiblock pattern (marked *X*) causing intermittent bifascicular block pattern. The degree of aberrant ventricular conduction varies intermittently.

The direct cause for the aberrant ventricular conduction is that the atrial premature impulse is conducted to the ventricles during a partial refractory period. However, the fundamental reason why aberrant ventricular conduction is almost a rule rather than exception during atrial bigeminy can be explained as follows. The ventricular cycle immediately preceding a given heart beat significantly influences the refractoriness of the cardiac conduction. In other words, the longer the ventricular cycle (R-R interval), the longer the refractory period following it; the shorter the ventricular cycle, the shorter the refractory period. This electrophysiologic property of the heart was described by Ashman in 1945, and this finding is called Ashman's phenomenon. The Ashman's phenomenon is responsible for frequent aberrant ventricular conduction in atrial bigeminy.

The striking ECG abnormality in this tracing is relatively tall R wave in lead V_1. This finding represents a true posterior myocardial infarction (see Chapter 3), which he had suffered 3 months previously.

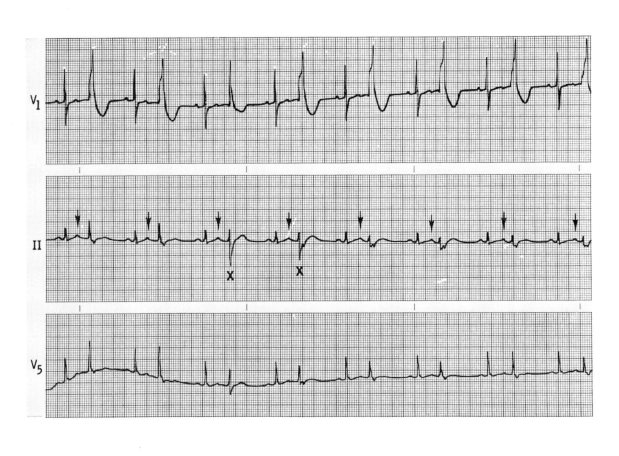

CASE 89

A 62-year-old man was admitted to the Intermediate Coronary Care Unit because of frequent episodes of palpitation. He stated that the palpitation was often initiated by emotional excitement or physical exercise.

1. What is your cardiac rhythm diagnosis?
2. What is the treatment of choice?

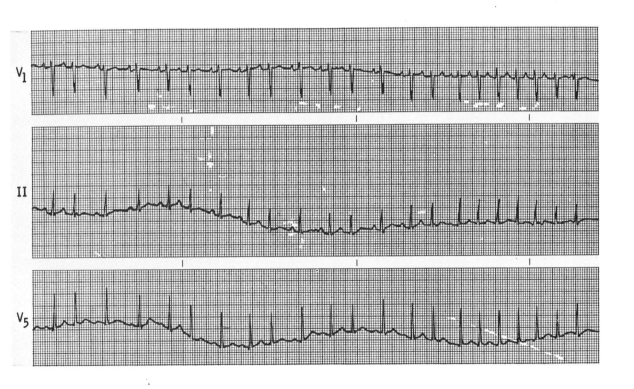

CASE 89: DIAGNOSIS

The underlying cardiac rhythm is sinus tachycardia with a rate of 110 beats per minute.

Note frequent atrial premature contractions which lead to paroxysmal atrial tachycardia with a rate of 180 beats per minute (the last portion of the tracing).

It has been well documented that paroxysmal atrial tachycardia is commonly initiated by frequent atrial premature contractions. The reason for this is that the same ectopic focus in the atria is capable of producing an isolated atrial premature contraction as well as atrial tachycardia. In addition, frequent atrial premature contractions may also lead to other atrial tachyarrhythmias including atrial flutter or fibrillation.

As far as the treatment is concerned, propranolol (Inderal) is considered to be the drug of choice for all types of catecholamine-induced tachyarrhythmias. Before treatment, however, possible underlying causes for atrial tachycardia should be investigated. The diagnostic tests for hyperthyroidism must be performed for every patient with atrial tachyarrhythmias because unexplainable atrial tachyarrhythmias are often due to hyperthyroidism. In addition, Wolff-Parkinson-White syndrome (see Chapter 11) should always be considered for a possible cause of palpitation in every case.

This patient failed to show any direct cause for the tachycardia.

CASE 90

The Holter monitor electrocardiogram was obtained from a 59-year-old woman with frequent episodes of palpitation. The routine electrocardiograms (12 leads) taken on many occasions failed to record any episode of ectopic tachyarrhythmias, although her resting heart rate has been rapid (rate 120–140 beats per minute).

The rhythm strips A, B, and C are not continuous.

1. *What is your cardiac rhythm diagnosis?*
2. *What is the most likely underlying disorder?*

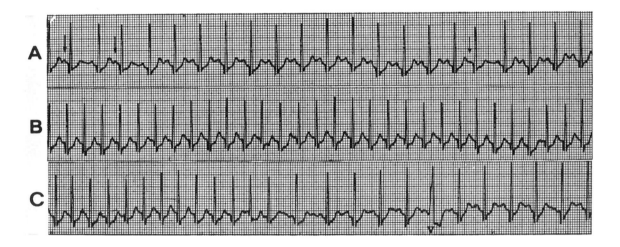

CASE 90: DIAGNOSIS

The underlying cardiac rhythm is sinus tachycardia with a rate of 138 beats per minute.

The Holter monitor ECG tracings documented paroxysmal atrial tachycardia (rate 200 beats per minute) initiated by atrial premature contractions (indicated by *arrows*). In addition, there is a ventricular premature contraction (marked *V*).

This patient was found to have hyperthyroidism. It is a well-known fact that sinus tachycardia even during a resting period is very common in patients with hyperthyroidism, and various atrial tachyarrhythmias are also frequently observed in this disease.

CASE 91

A 74-year-old man was brought to the emergency room because of palpitation associated with lightheadedness. He was not taking any drug.

1. *What is your cardiac rhythm diagnosis?*
2. *What should be done first?*

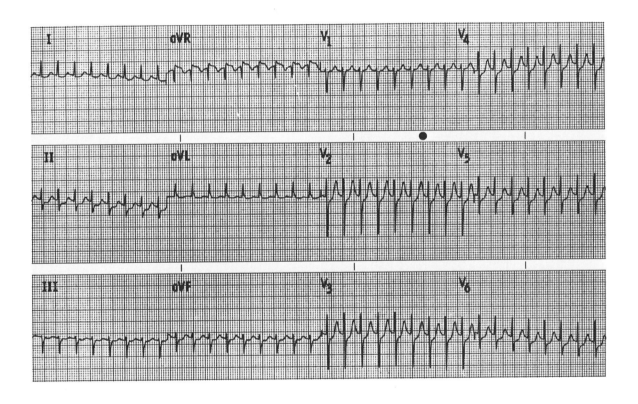

CASE 91: DIAGNOSIS

The rate is extremely rapid (rate 215 beats per minute), and the rhythm is precisely regular with normal QRS complexes, yet no P waves are discernible. This type of rapid heart action is termed "supraventricular tachycardia" because it is not possible to determine the exact origin of cardiac impulse formation. Since ventricular tachycardia can be excluded in view of normal QRS complexes, the term supraventricular tachycardia is used.

Supraventricular tachycardia is often a manifestation of reciprocating (re-entrant or circus-movement) tachycardia. On the other hand, supraventricular tachycardia may actually be paroxysmal atrial or A-V junctional tachycardia because P waves are often buried in the QRS complexes.

The best therapeutic approach, under this circumstance, is immediate application of carotid sinus stimulation, which was successful in terminating the tachycardia on this patient. If carotid sinus stimulation is ineffective, however, various other measures including direct current shock, intravenous injection of rapid-acting digitalis preparation (e.g., digoxin, Cedilanid, etc.) or propranolol (Inderal) should be tried depending on the clinical circumstance. After a restoration of sinus rhythm, many patients require an antiarrhythmic agent. Digitalis and propranolol (Inderal) are the most commonly used agents, and they are usually effective.

Diffuse S-T segment depression in many leads is primarily due to the rapid rate.

CASE 92

A 66-year-old man complained of nausea and vomiting preceded by a loss of appetite during rapid digitalization for acute congestive heart failure due to coronary heart disease.

What is your cardiac rhythm diagnosis?

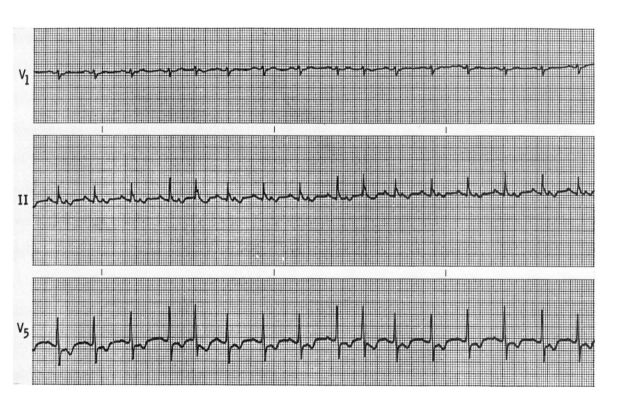

CASE 92: DIAGNOSIS

Arrows indicate ectopic P waves. The cardiac rhythm reveals atrial tachycardia (atrial rate 190 beats per minute) with varying Wenckebach A-V block and intermittent 2:1 A-V block. Under this circumstance, 2:1 A-V block is actually a variant of Wenckebach A-V block (see Case 131).

Atrial tachycardia with A-V block is often called "atrial tachycardia with block" or "PAT with block." This rhythm disorder is almost a pathognomonic feature of digitalis intoxication.

The T wave inversion in lead V₅ is a manifestation of lateral myocardial ischemia.

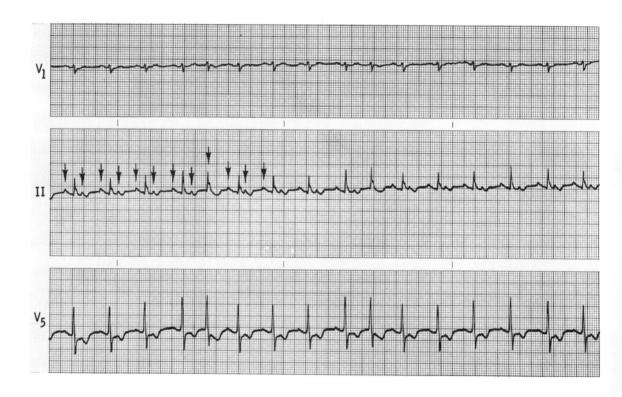

CASE 93

This electrocardiogram was obtained from a 77-year-old woman with chronic congestive heart failure due to hypertensive heart disease. Digitalis toxicity was suspected.

What is your cardiac rhythm diagnosis?

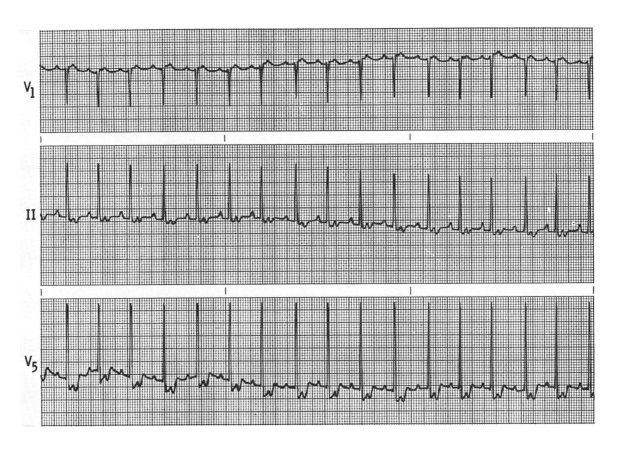

CASE 93: DIAGNOSIS

Arrows indicate ectopic P waves. The cardiac rhythm is atrial tachycardia (atrial rate 226 beats per minute, indicated by *arrows*) with 2:1 A-V block. Note that every other P wave is not followed by QRS complexes. The fact that atrial tachycardia with A-V block is almost always due to digitalis toxicity has been emphasized previously (see Case 92).

Note markedly increased QRS voltage in lead V₅ with secondary S-T, T wave changes indicative of left ventricular hypertrophy (see Case 10).

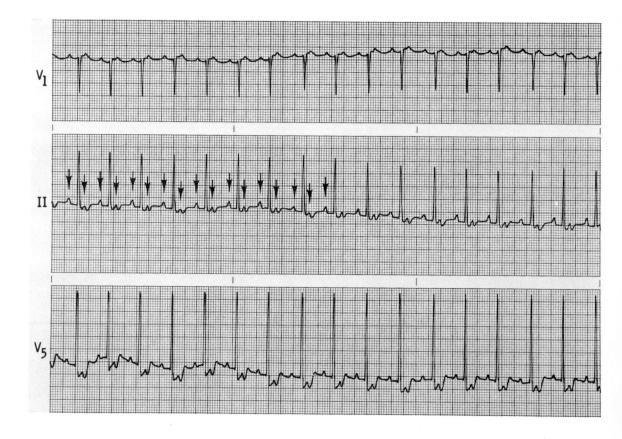

CASE 94

This electrocardiogram was obtained from an 86-year-old woman with chronic cor-pulmonale due to chronic obstructive pulmonary disease.

What is your cardiac rhythm diagnosis?

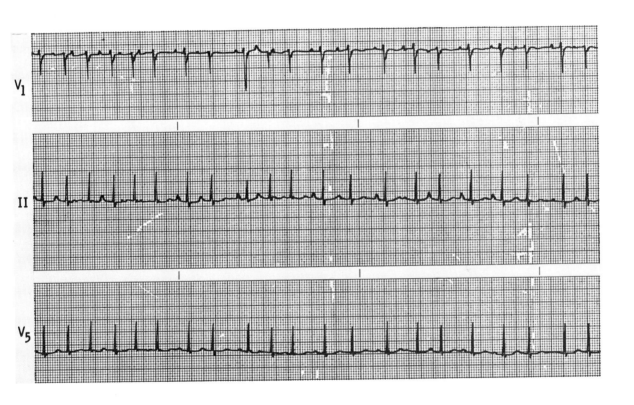

CASE 94: DIAGNOSIS

The cardiac rhythm is multifocal atrial tachycardia with rate ranging from 120–160 beats per minute. Note varying configurations of the P waves with varying P-P cycles as well as the P-R intervals. In addition, some QRS complexes are slightly bizarre because of aberrant ventricular conduction.

The diagnostic criteria of multifocal atrial tachycardia are as follows:

1. Two or more ectopic P waves with different configurations.
2. Two or more different ectopic P-P cycles.
3. Atrial rate between 100–250 beats per minute (occasionally slower than 100 beats per minute).
4. Isoelectric line present between P-P intervals.
5. Frequent occurrence of varying P-R intervals and A-V block of varying degree (nonconducted ectopic P waves).

The underlying disorder responsible for the production of multifocal atrial tachycardia is most commonly chronic cor-pulmonale as seen in this case. Less commonly, multifocal atrial tachycardia may be encountered in patients with pulmonary embolism, pneumonia, and hypoxia due to other various causes. This arrhythmia is occasionally observed postoperatively following various types of major surgery.

Note peaking and tall P waves indicative of P-pulmonale.

Multifocal atrial tachycardia has many other names such as chaotic atrial rhythm, chaotic atrial tachycardia, chaotic atrial mechanism, and malignant atrial tachycardia. As the names of this arrhythmia indicate, multifocal atrial tachycardia is difficult to treat. Various antiarrhythmic agents have little effect on this arrhythmia. Propranolol (Inderal) is effective in some cases with multifocal atrial tachycardia, providing that there is no contraindication. The improvement of the underlying pulmonary disease seems to be more beneficial than any antiarrhythmic drug for this arrhythmia in many cases. Occasionally, multifocal atrial tachycardia may transform to atrial fibrillation or flutter.

CASE 95

A 42-year-old hypertensive woman with chronic obstructive pulmonary disease was admitted to the hospital because of severe congestive heart failure.

What is your cardiac rhythm diagnosis?

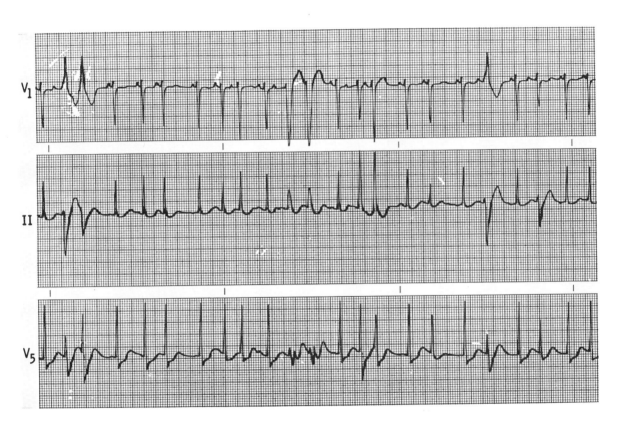

CASE 95: DIAGNOSIS

Arrows indicate ectopic P waves. The cardiac rhythm reveals multifocal atrial tachycardia with rate ranging from 130–165 beats per minute. The characteristic features of multifocal atrial tachycardia, including varying P wave configurations associated with varying P-P cycles as well as P-R intervals, are readily recognized (see Case 94).

In addition, there are frequent occurrences of aberrant ventricular conduction. It is interesting to note that some of the aberrantly conducted beats show right bundle branch block pattern (marked *R*), whereas others reveal left bundle branch block pattern (marked *L*). Furthermore, some aberrantly conducted beats exhibit left anterior hemiblock pattern (marked *X*) while others show a bifascicular block pattern consisting of right bundle branch block pattern and left anterior hemiblock pattern (marked *R* and *X*, respectively). These ECG findings are an excellent example of a *functional* trifascicular block (see Chapter 10). Ventricular premature contractions are closely simulated because of bizarre QRS complexes due to aberrant ventricular conduction.

The diagnosis of left ventricular hypertrophy can be made without any difficulty (see Case 10).

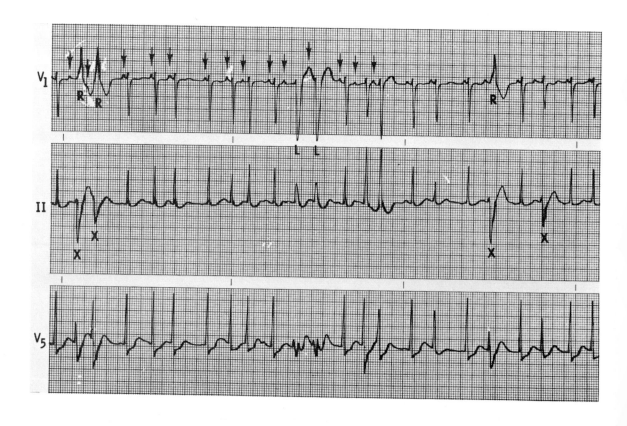

CASE 96

A 61-year-old man developed extremely rapid heart action postoperatively soon after gastrectomy (tracing A). Preoperatively, no definite evidence of heart disease was found. After restoration of sinus rhythm, another ECG tracing shown on the next page was obtained (tracing B).

   1. What is your cardiac rhythm diagnosis?
   2. What is the drug of choice?
   3. What other ECG abnormality is present?

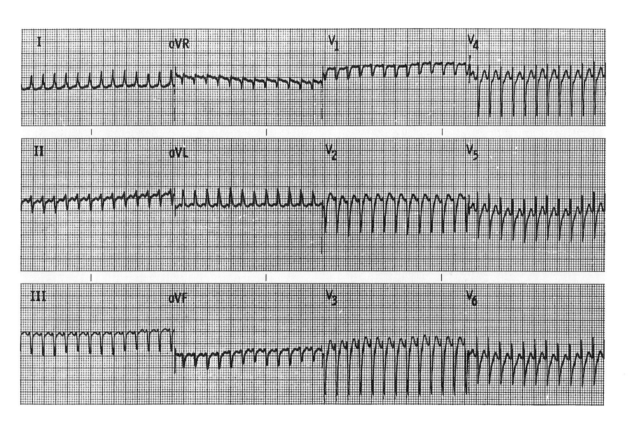

CASE 96: DIAGNOSIS

In tracing *A,* the heart rate is extremely rapid (rate 300 beats per minute), and the rhythm is precisely regular with normal QRS complexes. Thus, the cardiac rhythm diagnosis is atrial flutter with 1:1 A-V conduction. Whenever the heart rate is faster than 250 beats per minute and the rhythm is regular, the diagnosis of atrial flutter with 1:1 A-V conduction is certain.

In general, untreated atrial flutter almost always reveals 2:1 A-V conduction because the A-V junction has a longer defractory period than any portion of the heart (see Cases 97 and 98). Therefore, atrial flutter with 1:1 A-V conduction is extremely rare in older adults. When atrial flutter with 1:1 A-V conduction occurs, several possible underlying causes should be considered. They may include hyperthyroidism, Wolff-Parkinson-White syndrome (see Chapter 11), and quinidine effect. In addition, catecholamine-induced arrhythmia should always be considered under this circumstance.

In this patient, atrial flutter was considered to be catecholamine-induced, postoperatively. There was no other factor responsible for the production of this rapid heart action.

As repeatedly emphasized, the drug of choice for catecholamine-induced tachyarrhythmias is propranolol (Inderal). Intravenous injection of propranolol (Inderal) (2 mg) was effective in terminating atrial flutter in this case. In an urgent situation, however, particularly when propranolol is ineffective, immediate application of direct current shock will be the treatment of choice. Alternatively, parenteral rapid digitalization should be considered when proparnolol and direct current shock are ineffective.

Another ECG abnormality in tracing A is left anterior hemiblock (QRS axis −45°; see Chapter 10).

In tracing B, the underlying rhythm is marked sinus tachycardia with a rate of 160 beats per minute. There are frequent atrial premature contractions with aberrant ventricular conduction because of very short coupling intervals. It has been well documented that frequent atrial premature contractions are often preceded by and/or followed by paroxysmal atrial tachyarrhythmias (see also Cases 89 and 90).

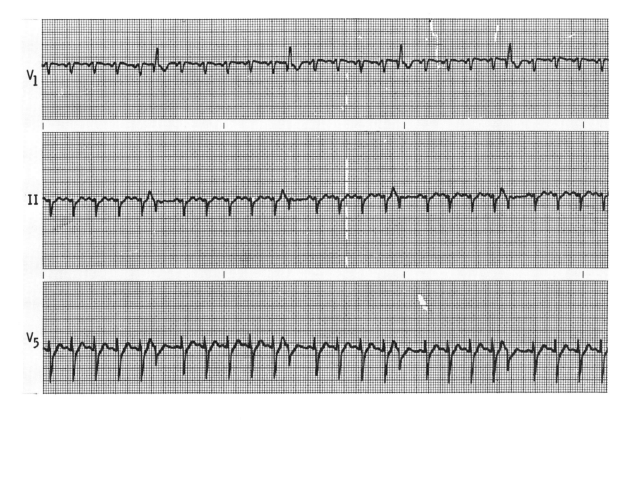

CASE 97

These cardiac rhythm strips were obtained from a 37-year-old black man with alcoholic cardiomyopathy. He was seen in the emergency room because of paroxysmal rapid heart action.

What is your cardiac rhythm diagnosis?

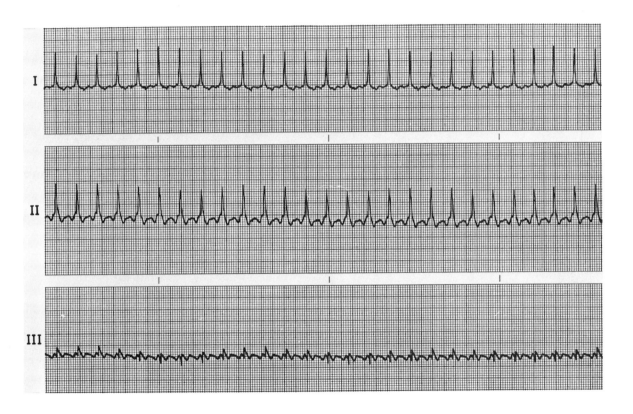

CASE 97: DIAGNOSIS

The cardiac rhythm reveals atrial flutter (atrial rate 320 beats per minute) with 2:1 A-V response. Note that every other flutter wave is not followed by QRS complexes.

It can be said that atrial flutter with 2:1 A-V response is one of the most common tachyarrhythmias seen in our daily practice. Yet, it is often misdiagnosed as other arrhythmias such as A-V junctional tachycardia, supraventricular tachycardia, or even sinus tachycardia when the flutter waves are not recognized.

In atrial flutter with 2:1 A-V response, the term "response" is used instead of "block," because 2:1 A-V conduction in atrial flutter is merely a physiologic rather than pathologic phenomenon. When the term "A-V block" is used, it implies an abnormally prolonged refractory period in the A-V junction. Thus, atrial flutter with 2:1 A-V *response* is the correct expression.

CASE 98

The ECG tracings shown on this page (tracing A) and on the next page (tracing B) were obtained from a 55-year-old man with chronic cor-pulmonale due to chronic obstructive pulmonary disease. He was admitted to the Coronary Care Unit because of advanced congestive heart failure associated with rapid heart action (tracing A). Tracing B was taken after treatment.

1. What is your cardiac rhythm diagnosis of tracing A?
2. What is the treatment of choice?
3. What is the other ECG abnormality?

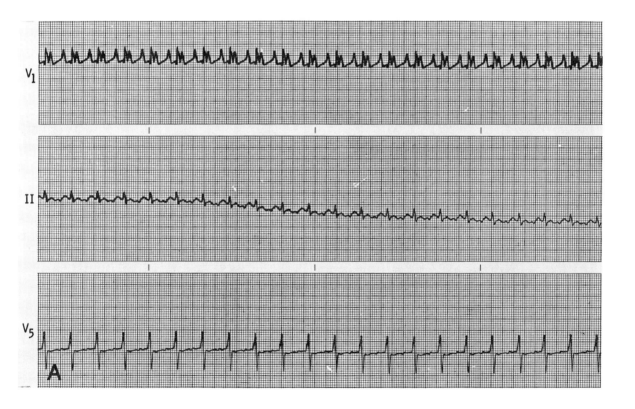

CASE 98: DIAGNOSIS

The cardiac rhythm shows atrial flutter (atrial rate 260 beats per minute) with 2:1 A-V response. Note that every other flutter wave is not conducted to the ventricles.

The treatment of choice for any supraventricular tachyarrhythmias including atrial flutter associated with congestive heart failure is rapid digitalization. Digitalis is extremely effective under this circumstance.

Tracing B, taken after digitalization reveals normal sinus rhythm with a rate of 85 beats per minute.

The striking abnormality in both ECG tracings is a tall R wave in lead V_1 due to right ventricular hypertrophy (see Case 12). In addition, right atrial enlargement (P-pulmonale) is also diagnosed (see Case 18). Peaked and tall flutter waves in lead V_1 represent right atrial enlargement (tracing A).

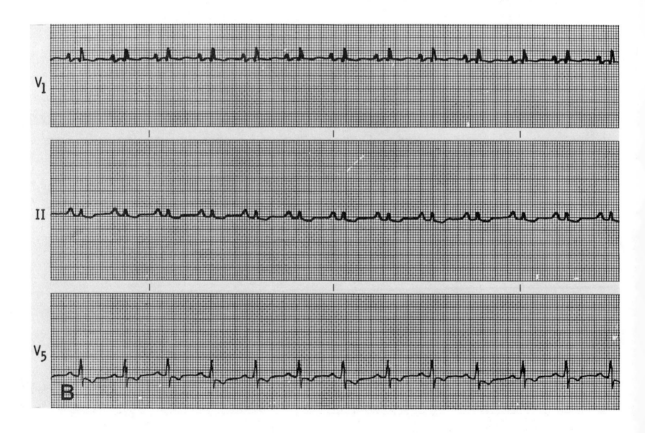

CASE 99

These cardiac rhythm strips were obtained from a 52-year-old man with chronic cor-pulmonale and hypertensive heart disease. He has been digitalized and quinidinized.

What is your cardiac rhythm diagnosis?

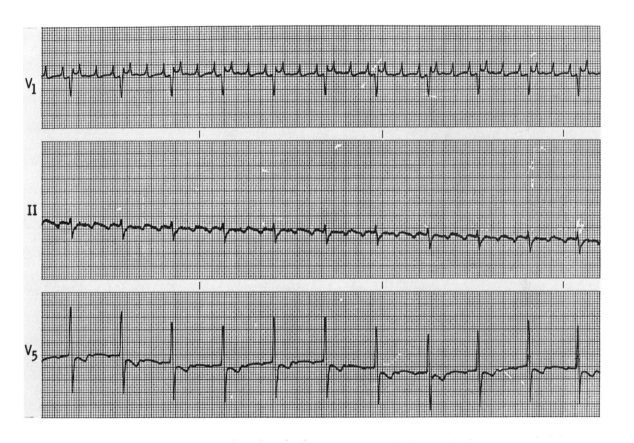

CASE 99: DIAGNOSIS

The cardiac rhythm reveals atrial flutter (atrial rate 219 beats per minute) with 3:1 A-V block. Note that every third flutter wave is conducted to the ventricles. In other words, the R-R interval shows three times the atrial flutter cycles. Atrial flutter with 3:1 A-V block is a rather uncommon conduction ratio. Under this circumstance, concealed A-V conduction is considered to be responsible.

Another interesting finding in this tracing is slower-than-usual atrial flutter (usual flutter rate 250–350 beats per minute). This slow flutter rate is a characteristic feature of quinidine effect (see also Case 103). It should be remembered that quinidine causes a prolonged refractoriness in the atria. On the other hand, digitalis produces the exact opposite phenomenon—namely, a shortening of the refractory period in the atria leading to acceleration of the atrial flutter cycles (see Case 106).

The peaked and tall flutter waves in lead V₁ represent right atrial hypertrophy. In addition, there is left anterior hemiblock because of left axis deviation of the QRS complexes (see Chapter 10). Left ventricular hypertrophy is also suggested.

CASE 100

These cardiac rhythm strips were obtained from a 64-year-old man with coronary and hypertensive heart disease. He has been taking digoxin (0.25 mg) and hydrochlorothiazide (25 mg) daily for several months.

1. *What is your cardiac rhythm diagnosis?*
2. *What is the ECG abnormality?*

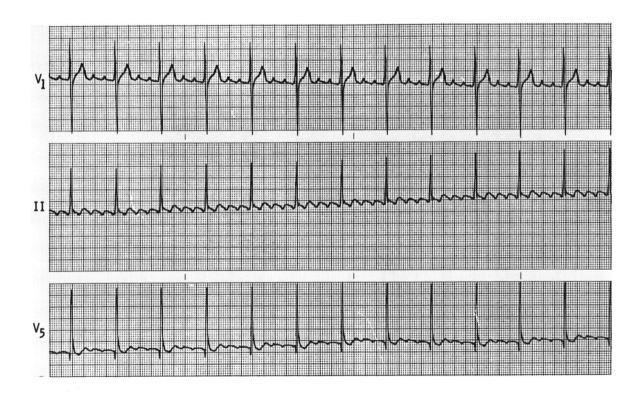

CASE 100: DIAGNOSIS

Cardiac rhythm discloses atrial flutter (atrial rate 300 beats per minute) with 4:1 A-V block. Note that every fourth flutter wave is conducted to the ventricles. The 4:1 A-V ratio means that the A-V conduction is abnormally prolonged as a result of digitalis effect. Thus, the term "block" is used and not "response." As mentioned earlier, atrial flutter with 2:1 A-V *response* is a physiologic phenomenon, and therefore 2:1 conduction in this case is *not* a block.

When the patient with atrial flutter with 2:1 A-V response is treated with digitalis, the rhythm often changes to atrial flutter with 4:1 A-V block as seen in this case. On other other hand, atrial flutter may transform to atrial fibrillation or even sinus rhythm may be restored by digitalization. Occasionally, the atrial flutter cycles may be accelerated by the digitalis (see Case 106).

It should be remembered that atrial flutter with 4:1 A-V block is *not* a manifestation of digitalis toxicity. However, atrial flutter with higher degree (5:1 or more A-V ratio) A-V block nearly always represents digitalis intoxication.

Note that the R wave is relatively tall in lead V_1 due to posterior myocardial infarction which had occurred 6 months previously. In addition, left ventricular hypertrophy is strongly suspected (see Case 10).

CASE 101

An 89-year-old man with chronic congestive heart failure due to coronary heart disease has been taking digoxin (0.25 mg) daily for 5 days a week.

What is your cardiac rhythm diagnosis?

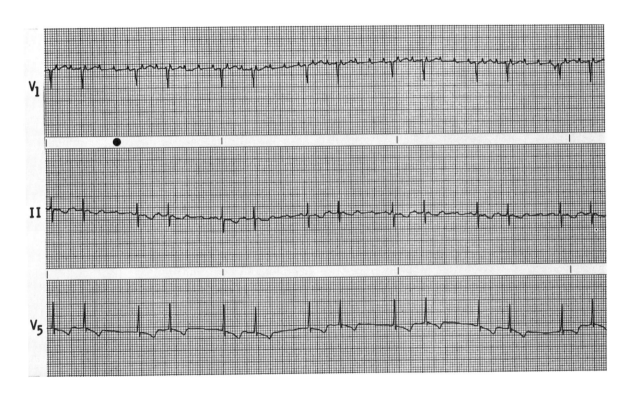

CASE 101: DIAGNOSIS

Cardiac rhythm reveals atrial flutter (atrial rate 260 beats per minute) with Wenckebach A-V response. The Wenckebach A-V response consists of alternating 4:1 and 2:1 A-V ratios causing a form of ventricular bigeminy (ventricular pseudo-bigeminy).

Wenckebach A-V response is diagnosed on the basis of a progressive lengthening of the F-R interval until a pause occurs. In addition, the long R-R interval is shorter than two short R-R intervals. Furthermore, the short R-R interval is longer than two atrial flutter cycles, whereas the long R-R interval is shorter than four flutter cycles. These ECG findings are the characteristic features of Wenckebach A-V response (see Case 131).

There is left axis deviation, and the inverted T wave in lead V_5 is suggestive of lateral myocardial ischemia.

CASE 102

These cardiac rhythm strips were obtained from a 56-year-old woman with mild congestive heart failure due to hypertensive heart disease.

What is your cardiac rhythm diagnosis?

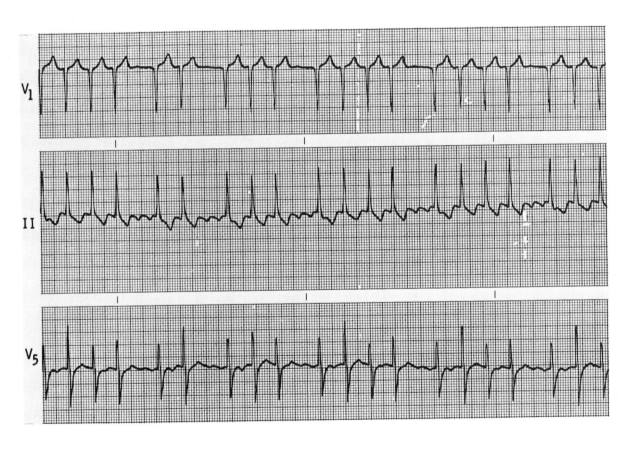

CASE 102: DIAGNOSIS

The cardiac rhythm is atrial flutter (atrial rate 320 beats per minute) with varying Wenckebach A-V response. The diagnosis of Wenckebach A-V response can be made without any difficulty on the basis of a progressive shortening of the R-R intervals until a pause occurs (see Case 131). The progressive increment of the F-R intervals which is a characteristic feature of Wenckebach A-V response can not be determined readily in this tracing since the flutter waves are not clearly evident in some areas. This is, of course, due to the fact that their superimposition to other segment of ECG complexes.

In a practical sense, Wenckebach phenomenon should be considered as the first possible diagnosis when dealing with group beats followed by a pause.

Wenckebach phenomenon has been described elsewhere (see Case 131).

It should be noted that some QRS complexes are slightly bizarre, particularly following long ventricular pauses. These bizarre QRS complexes represent aberrant ventricular conduction due to Ashman's phenomenon (see Case 88).

CASE 103

This ECG tracing was obtained from a 58-year-old man with hypertensive heart disease.

1. *What is your cardiac rhythm diagnosis?*
2. *What cardiac drug(s) is (are) responsible for this cardaic rhythm disorder?*

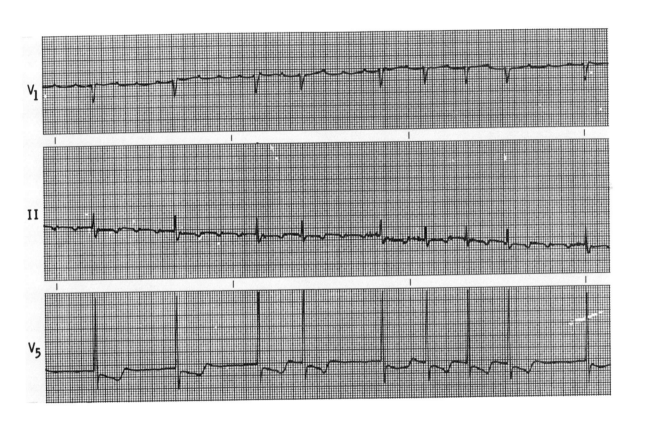

CASE 103: DIAGNOSIS

The cardiac rhythm discloses atrial flutter (atrial rate 175 beats per minute) with varying Wenckebach A-V response and intermittent 4:1 A-V block (see Case 131).

Obviously, the flutter cycle is much slower than usual (usual atrial flutter rate 250–350 beats per minute). Yet, two components (saw-tooth appearance) of the flutter wave, the characteristic feature of atrial flutter, are clearly evident. As mentioned previously, a unique electrophysiologic property of quinidine is to reduce the atrial flutter rate by increasing the refrectory period in the atria.

Another drug he has been taking is digoxin which is responsible for slow ventricular rate as a result of increased A-V block.

He has been taking digoxin (0.25 mg) once and quinidine (0.3 gm) 4 times daily in the hope that the sinus rhythm may be restored.

The diagnosis of left ventricular hypertrophy is obvious (see Case 10).

CASE 104

These cardiac rhythm strips were obtained from a 60-year-old man with idiopathic cardiomyopathy.

What is your cardiac rhythm diagnosis?

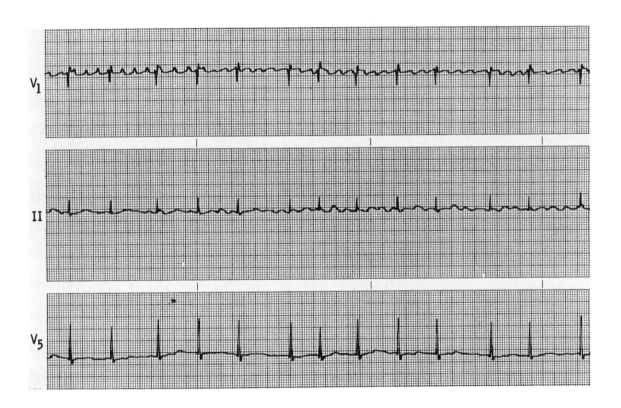

CASE 104: DIAGNOSIS

The cardiac rhythm is an atypical form of atrial flutter (atrial rate 300–325 beats per minute) with varying degree A-V block. It should be noted that the atrial flutter cycles are not only irregular, but also the configuration of the flutter waves varies.

It has been reported that this type of atypical atrial flutter is not uncommonly encountered in patients with caridomyopathy. In addition, quinidine occasionally causes the atypical atrial flutter as shown in this ECG tracing.

The fundamental mechanism responsible for the production of this atypical atrial flutter is uncertain. Nevertheless, the finding is probably due to uneven circus movement (re-entrant cycle) of the atrial flutter waves.

This patient has been taking digoxin and quinidine.

CASE 105

This ECG tracing was obtained from a 10-year-old girl postoperatively for the transposition of the great vessels. This slow rhythm had persisted after the operation.

What is your cardiac rhythm diagnosis?

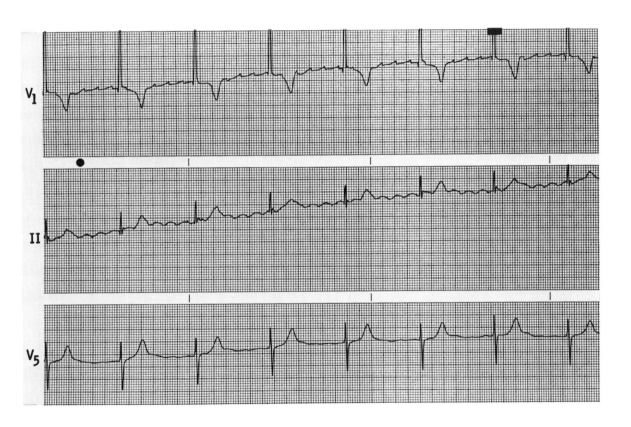

CASE 105: DIAGNOSIS

The cardiac rhythm reveals atrial flutter (atrial rate 280 beats per minute) with A-V junctional escape rhythm (ventricular rate 48 beats per minute) due to complete A-V block. Note that none of the atrial flutter impulses are conducted to the ventricles so that the A-V junctional pacemaker controls the ventricular activity independently resulting in complete A-V dissociation (see Chapter 7). The F-R distance (the distance from the last flutter wave to the next QRS complex) varies throughout, but the R-R intervals are precisely regular indicating independency between the atria and the ventricles.

In general, when the A-V conduction ratio appears to be more than 4:1 in atrial flutter, complete A-V block is almost always present.

Note a tall R wave in lead V_1 indicative of severe right ventricular hypertrophy.

This child required a permanent artificial pacemaker implantation.

CASE 106

A 62-year-old man with rheumatic heart disease was admitted to the hospital because of acute congestive heart failure associated with rapid heart action. He was digitalized with marked improvement. This ECG tracing was taken several days after digitalization started.

What is your cardiac rhythm diagnosis?

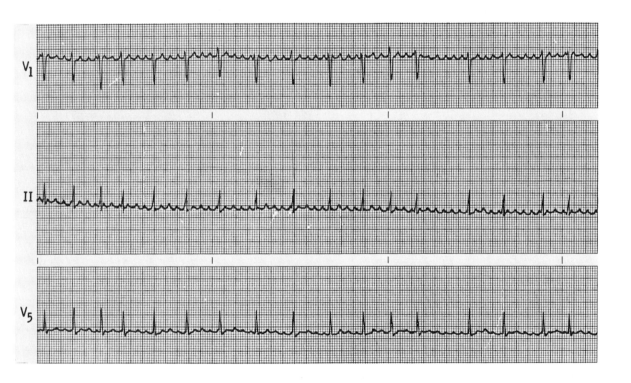

CASE 106: DIAGNOSIS

The cardiac rhythm exhibits atrial impure flutter (atrial rate 400 beats per minute) with varying A-V response. The term "atrial impure flutter" is used when the atrial flutter rate is more than 350 beats (usual rate range 350–450 beats per minute) per minute. As described previously, the usual uncomplicated atrial flutter has rate ranging from 250–350 beats per minute (see Cases 97 and 100).

In this patient, the atrial rate was accelerated by digitalization because the drug shortens the refractory period in the atria. The pretreatment atrial flutter rate in this case was 320 beats per minute.

It is a well-known fact that atrial flutter or fibrillation is common in patients with rheumatic heart disease. After digitalization, a restoration of sinus rhythm is often accomplished in many patients with rheumatic heart disease.

CASE 107

A 54-year-old man was admitted to the Coronary Care Unit because of acute congestive heart failure associated with extremely rapid heart rate. He was not taking any drug on admission.

What is your cardiac rhythm diagnosis?

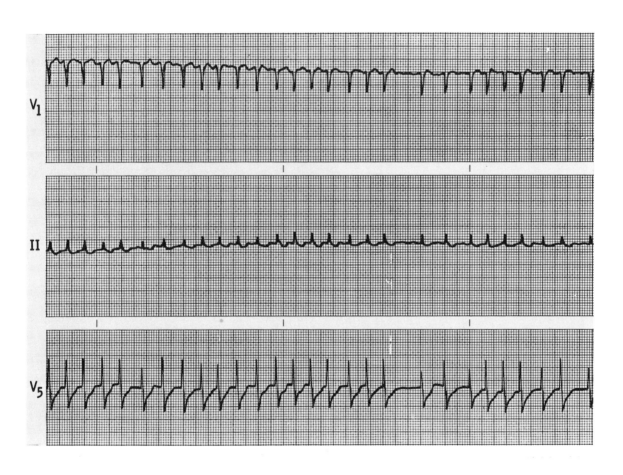

CASE 107: DIAGNOSIS

The cardiac rhythm reveals atrial fibrillation with a very rapid ventricular response (ventricular rate 160–250 beats per minute). In some portions of the tracing, the R-R intervals appear to be regular because the maximal numbers of the atrial impulses are conducted to the ventricles.

He was rapidly digitalized. This patient improved markedly by digitalization with diuretic therapy, and sinus rhythm was restored. In general, the efficacy of digitalis preparation is most striking when patients suffer from acute congestive heart failure associated with atrial fibrillation with a very rapid ventricular response as seen in this case.

CASE 108

These cardiac rhythm strips were obtained from an 89-year-old woman with acute congestive heart failure due to hypertensive heart disease.

What is your cardiac rhythm diagnosis?

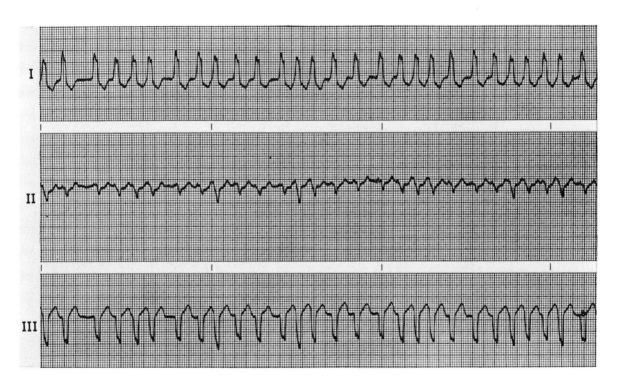

CASE 108: DIAGNOSIS

The cardiac rhythm shows atrial fibrillation associated with left bundle branch block with a very rapid ventricular response (ventricular rate 170–200 beats per minute). Ventricular tachycardia is closely simulated because of rapid ventricular rate, and bizarre and broad QRS complexes. However, ventricular tachycardia is definitely excluded on the basis of a grossly irregular ventricular cycle. In elderly individuals, atrial fibrillatory waves are usually not clearly evident and this finding is termed "fine atrial fibrillation" to distinguish it from "coarse" atrial fibrillation (the amplitude of fibrillatory wave being more than 1 mm; see Case 110).

As far as the underlying disease is concerned, a fine atrial fibrillation is usually due to coronary and/or hypertensive heart disease, whereas a coarse atrial fibrillation is nearly always found in patients with rheumatic heart disease, particularly mitral stenosis (see Case 110). Less commonly a coarse atrial fibrillation may be found in patients with hyperthyroidism.

She was rapidly digitalized with marked improvement.

CASE 109

This ECG tracing was obtained from an 82-year-old man with advanced congestive heart failure due to coronary heart disease. He was not taking any drug.

1. What is your cardiac rhythm diagnosis?
2. What is the other ECG abnormality?

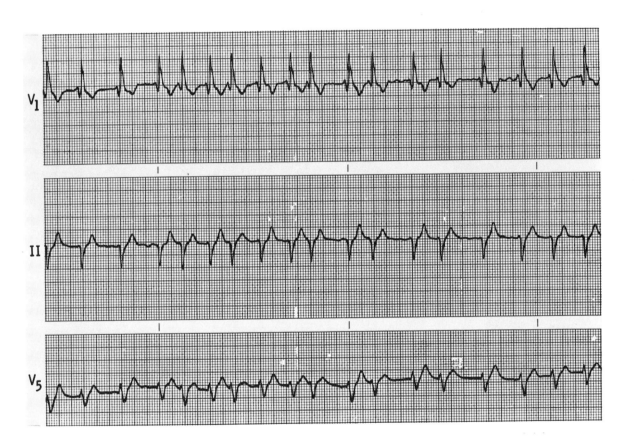

CASE 109: DIAGNOSIS

The cardiac rhythm is atrial fibrillation associated with right bundle branch block with a rapid ventricular response (ventricular rate 110–160 beats per minute). Again, ventricular tachycardia is superficially simulated because of a rapid ventricular rate with bizarre and broad QRS complexes. Grossly irregular ventricular cycle is a key factor to exclude a possibility of ventricular tachycardia.

Another ECG abnormality is marked left axis deviation (QRS axis −60°, calculated from a 12-lead ECG) which represents left anterior hemiblock. Thus, this patient has a bifascicular block (incomplete bilateral bundle branch block) consisting of right bundle branch block and left anterior hemiblock (see Chapter 10).

In addition, lateral myocardial infarction is strongly suspected because of a small Q wave with a markedly reduced R wave amplitude in lead V_5. In fact, he had suffered from myocardial infarction 3 months previously.

CASE 110

This ECG tracing was obtained from a 53-year-old man who has been taking digoxin (0.25 mg) daily for several years.

1. *What is your cardiac rhythm diagnosis?*
2. *Which cardiac chamber(s) is (are) enlarged?*
3. *What is most likely his underlying heart disease?*

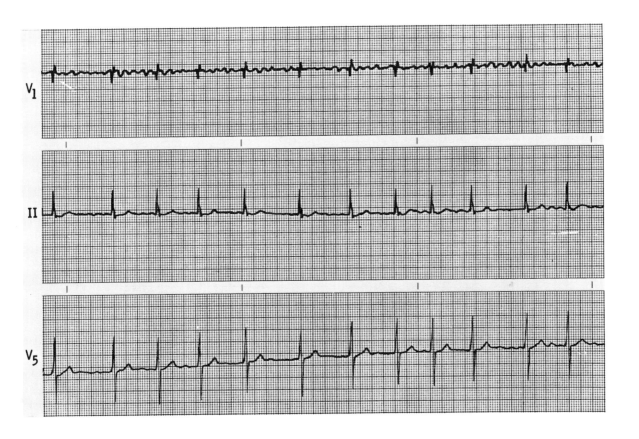

CASE 110: DIAGNOSIS

The cardiac rhythm is a coarse atrial fibrillation. Note that the amplitude of the fibrillatory waves is large (fibrillatory amplitude more than 1 mm), particularly in lead V_1. The ventricular rate is ideally maintained (rate 70–85 beats per minute) in this patient by a maintenance digitalis therapy.

Coarse atrial fibrillation is almost always (more than 75%) encountered in patients with rheumatic heart disease, especially mitral stenosis, which this patient has. In addition, coarse atrial fibrillatory waves usually indicate significant left atrial hypertrophy (see Case 11).

Another ECG abnormality is RR' in lead V_1 (incomplete right bundle branch block *pattern*), and this finding represents right ventricular hypertrophy (see Case 12).

In summary, this ECG tracing shows typical findings diagnostic for rheumatic mitral stenosis.

CASE 111

A 59-year-old woman was admitted to the Coronary Care Unit because of severe chest pain of a few hours' duration. She was not taking any drug.

1. *What is your cardiac rhythm diagnosis?*
2. *What is the other ECG abnormality?*

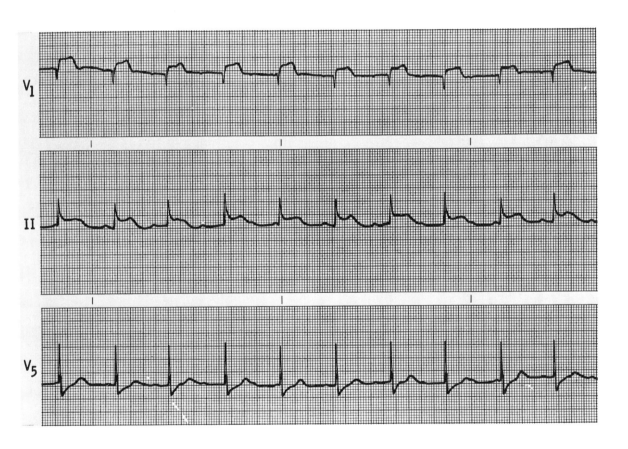

CASE 111: DIAGNOSIS

Arrows indicate ectopic P waves. The cardiac rhythm is atrial tachycardia (atrial rate 165 beats per minute, indicated by *arrows*) with independent nonparoxysmal A-V junctional tachycardia (ventricular rate 70 beats per minute) causing complete A-V dissociation (see Chapter 7). It should be noted that the atrial and ventricular activity is entirely independent. As a result, there are double supraventricular tachyarrhythmias.

It has been well documented that every known type of cardiac arrhythmia may be observed in patients with acute myocardial infarction, particularly during the first 24–72 hours. Nonparoxysmal A-V junctional tachycardia (see Chapter 7) is extremely common in acute diaphragmatic (inferior) myocardial infarction, because a blood supply to the A-V junction is impaired.

Another ECG abnormality is an elevation of S-T segment in leads II and V₁ (complete ECG shows S-T segment elevation in leads II, III, aVF, and V₁ through V₃) due to diaphragmatic and anteroseptal subepicardial injury (see Chapter 3) which is usually a manifestation of an early change in acute myocardial infarction. Within several hours after admission, a full-blown picture of acute diaphragmatic and anteroseptal myocardial infarction is documented on this patient.

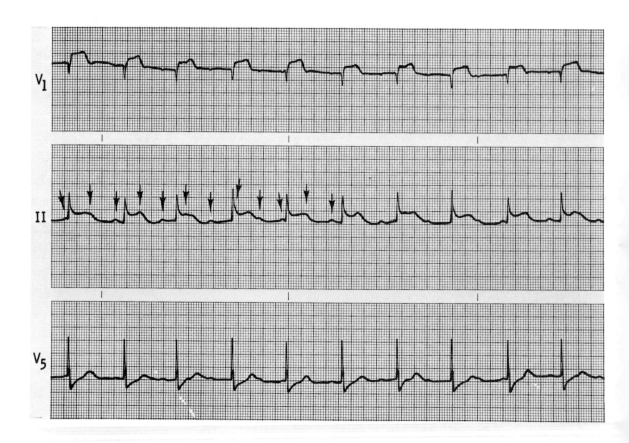

chapter 7

ATRIOVENTRICULAR (A-V) JUNCTIONAL ARRHYTHMIAS

CASE 112

This electrocardiogram was obtained from a 69-year-old man with carcinoma of the esophagus.

What is your cardiac rhythm diagnosis?

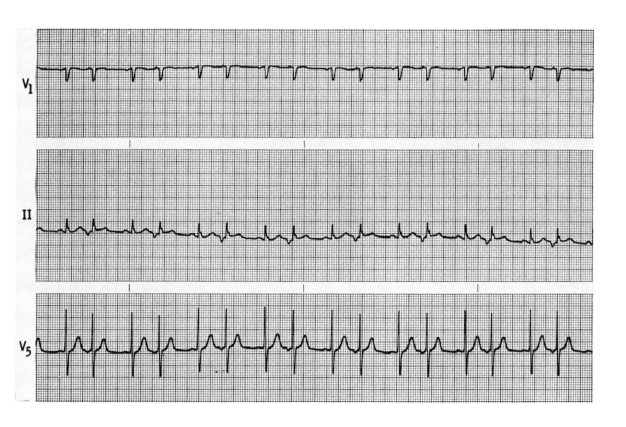

CASE 112: DIAGNOSIS

Arrows indicate ectopic P waves. The underlying cardiac rhythm is sinus tachycardia with a rate of 105 beats per minute. There are frequent A-V junctional premature contractions (indicated by *arrows*) which occur on every other beat, producing A-V junctional bigeminy.

Note that the ectopic P waves (indicated by *arrows*) are conducted in a retrograde fashion to the atria (inverted P waves in lead II), and the P-R interval is short. It should be stressed that the P-R interval in A-V junctional beat is a difference between antegrade (forward) conduction time from the A-V junctional pacemaker to the ventricles and the retrograde conduction time from the A-V junctional pacemaker to the atria. In other words, the P-R interval in the A-V junctional beat is *not* an expression of the usual A-V conduction sequence as seen in sinus beats or atrial premature beats. Thus, the P-R interval of the uncomplicated A-V junctional beat (either A-V junctional premature beats, A-V junctional escape beats, or A-V junctional tachycardia) is usually shorter than 0.12 second (see also Case 115).

In A-V junctional beats, the inverted P waves may be preceded by or followed by QRS complexes depending on the sequence of atrial and ventricular activation. That is, the atria may be activated by the A-V junctional pacemaker before the ventricular activation or vice versa. In addition, the P waves may be absent when the atria and the ventricles are activated by the A-V junctional pacemaker simultaneously so that the inverted P waves will be superimposed on the QRS complexes (see Cases 114 and 121).

In the A-V junctional beats, however, the P-R interval may be prolonged (longer than 0.12 second) when a significant antegrade conduction delay is present. On the other hand, the R-P interval will be prolonged (even longer than 0.20 second) when there is a prolonged retrograde conduction (see Case 126).

At present, the customary terms, "upper nodal," "mid-nodal," or "lower nodal," judged merely from the atrial and ventricular activation sequence (*e.g.,* "upper nodal" was used when the P wave preceded the QRS complex; "lower nodal" was used when the QRS complex preceded the P wave, and "mid-nodal" was used when there was no P wave), have been completely abandoned, because it is impossible to determine the exact location of the A-V junctional pacemaker from the P-R and R-P relationships. For a similar reason, the term "A-V *junctional*" replaced the old term "A-V *nodal.*"

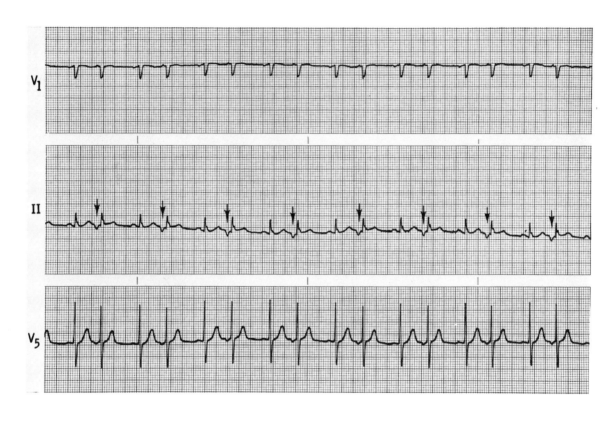

CASE 113

A 52-year-old man was brought to the emergency room because of palpitation. He was not taking any cardiac drug.

What is your cardiac rhythm diagnosis?

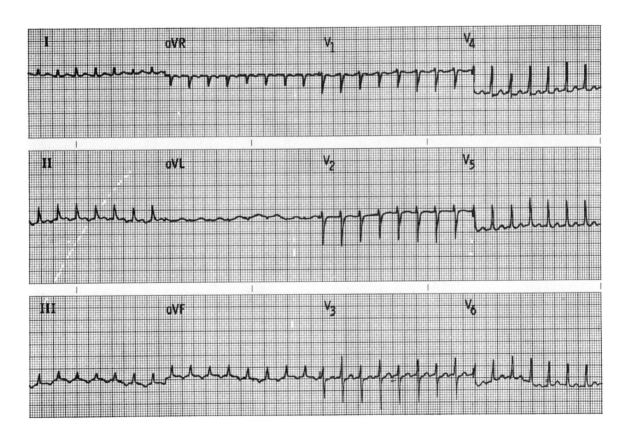

CASE 113: DIAGNOSIS

The cardiac rhythm reveals paroxysmal A-V junctional tachycardia with a rate of 187 beats per minute. Note inverted P waves which precede the QRS complexes.

Atrioventricular junctional tachycardia is classified into two types: paroxysmal and nonparoxysmal. In paroxysmal A-V junctional tachycardia as seen in this case, the onset and termination of the tachycardia are usually abrupt as the name designates and the rate is fast (rate 160–250 beats). The clinical significance of and the therapeutic approach to the paroxysmal A-V junctional tachycardia are the same as for paroxysmal atrial tachycardia (see Chapter 6, Cases 89 and 90).

On the other hand, nonparoxysmal A-V junctional tachycardia often persists as long as the underlying cause is not corrected, and it is *not* paroxysmal in nature. The usual rate of the nonparoxysmal A-V junctional tachycardia is much slower (rate 70–130 beats per minute; see Cases 115–121) than the paroxysmal form. Clinically, nonparoxysmal A-V junctional tachycarida is most commonly found in digitalis intoxication (see Cases 116–119), and less commonly it is encountered in acute diaphragmatic myocardial infarction (see Case 120) and following major surgery (see Case 121).

Carotid sinus stimulation is often effective in terminating paroxysmal A-V junctional tachycardia. Digitalis and propranolol (Inderal) are equally effective. Needless to say, possible causes such as excessive use of coffee, tea, or Coca-Cola, heavy smoking, hyperthyroidism, Wolff-Parkinson-White syndrome, mitral valve prolapse syndrome, myocarditis or pericarditis, and any other organic heart diseases should be investigated for every patient with unexplainable ectopic tachyarrhythmias.

Note that the QRS amplitude is low (low voltage, see Case 32), and this patient was found to have pericardial effusion due to malignancy. Slight variation of the QRS configuration in some leads is suggestive of 2:1 ventricular electrical alternans (see lead V_3) which is again common in pericardial effusion. In addition, the S-T segment is slightly but diffusely elevated, and the finding is compatible with acute pericarditis (see Chapter 4).

CASE 114

A 69-year-old man was brought to the emergency room because of rapid heart action associated with mild congestive heart failure. He was not taking any drug. The ECG tracing
shown on this page was taken on admission (tracing A), while another ECG taken on the
following day after treatment is shown on the next page (tracing B).

What is your cardiac rhythm diagnosis?

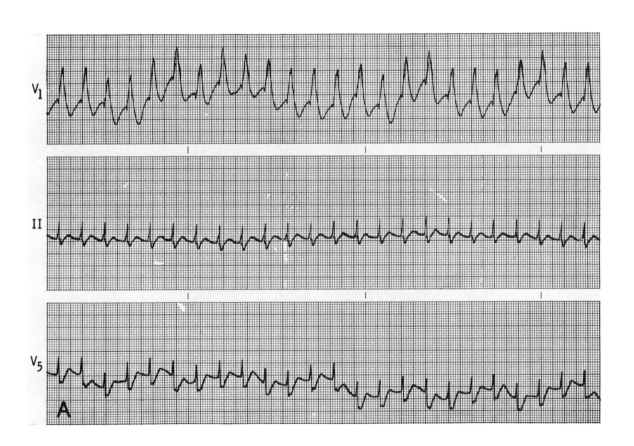

CASE 114: DIAGNOSIS

In tracing A, the QRS complexes are broad and bizarre with no P waves, and the rhythm is precisely regular with a rate of 160 beats per minute. When dealing with this type of tachycardia, it is not absolutely certain whether it represents ventricular tachycardia or supraventricular tachycardia with bundle branch block or aberrant ventricular conduction.

To confirm the cardiac rhythm diagnosis, a comparison of the QRS configuration during tachycardia and during sinus rhythm is extremely important when the previous ECG tracings on the same patient are available. That is, a knowledge of the pre-existing right or left bundle branch block during sinus rhythm is the determining factor in the diagnosis of supraventricular tachycardia when the QRS morphology is identical during ectopic tachycardia and during sinus rhythm.

In this patient, the right bundle branch block is the pre-existing ECG abnormality during sinus rhythm (tracing B), and many ECG tracings taken previously showed the same finding. Thus, the diagnosis of supraventricular, most likely paroxysmal, A-V junctional tachycardia (rate 160 beats per minute) with right bundle branch block is confirmed (tracing A).

Tracing B shows normal sinus rhythm (rate 64 beats per minute) and right blunde branch block. After digitalization, sinus rhythm was restored in this patient.

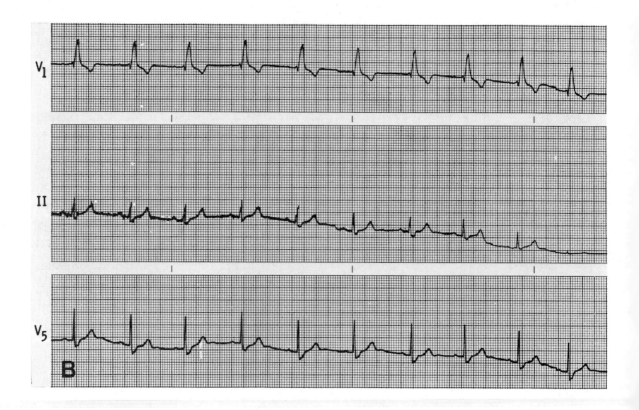

CASE 115

This ECG tracing was obtained from a 60-year-old man following abdominal aneurysmectomy. He has been taking quinidine (0.3 gm) 4 times daily for frequent ventricular premature contractions even before surgery.

1. What is your cardiac rhythm diagnosis?
2. What other ECG abnormality is present?

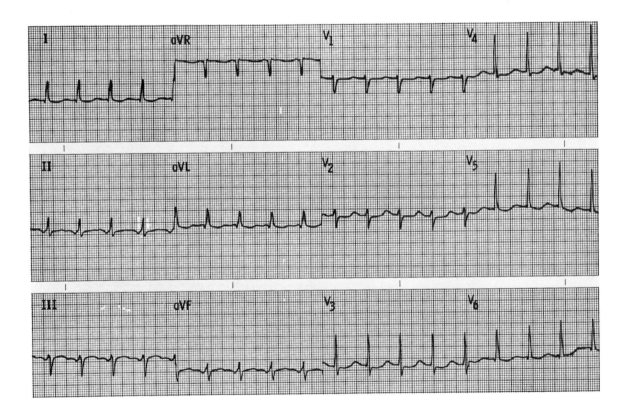

CASE 115: DIAGNOSIS

The cardiac rhythm is nonparoxysmal A-V junctional tachycardia with a rate of 103 beats per minute. Note that every QRS complex is preceded by a retrograde P wave (inverted P waves in leads II, III, and aVF, and upright P waves in lead aVR) with a short P-R interval.

As indicated previously (see Case 113), nonparoxysmal A-V junctional tachycardia is not uncommon following any major surgery, either cardiac or noncardiac. Postoperative hypoxia is considered to be responsible for the production of nonparoxysmal A-V junctional tachycardia under this circumstance.

It should be recognized that the Q-T interval is prolonged as a result of quinidine effect. In addition, there are nonspecific S-T, T wave abnormalities.

CASE 116

These cardiac rhythm strips were obtained from a 70-year-old man with chronic congestive heart failure due to hypertensive heart disease. Digitalis intoxication was suspected.

What is your cardiac rhythm diagnosis?

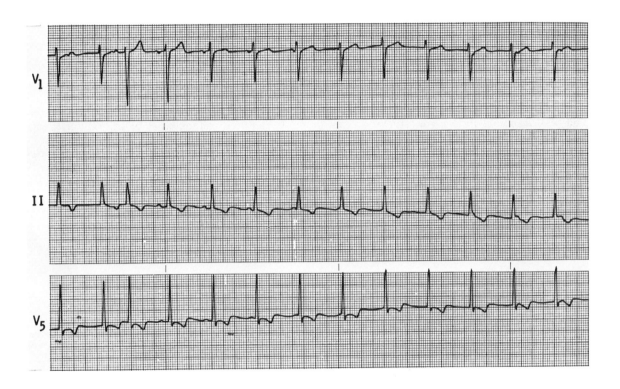

CASE 116: DIAGNOSIS

Arrows indicate sinus P waves. The cardiac rhythm discloses sinus rhythm (indicated by *arrows*, atrial rate 78 beats per minute) with nonparoxysmal A-V junctional tachycardia (ventricular rate 80 beats per minute) producing incomplete A-V dissociation. Note two ventricular captured beats (conducted sinus beats, marked *CB*) with slight aberrant ventricular conduction.

The term "A-V dissociation" is used when the atria and ventricles beat independently. A-V dissociation is an end result of some other underlying cardiac rhythm disorders which include:

1. Slowing of the sinus rate.
2. Acceleration of the A-V junctional or ventricular impulse formation.
3. Failure of the supraventricular impulses to reach the ventricles (*e.g.*, S-A block or A-V block).
4. Artificial (ventricular) pacemaker induced ventricular rhythm.
5. Combinations of the above.

The term "complete" A-V dissociation is used when the atrial and ventricular activities are independent throughout (see Cases 117–120). On the other hand, the term "incomplete" A-V dissociation is used when the atria and the ventricles become related even momentarily. In other words, incomplete A-V dissociation is diagnosed when one or more captured (either atrial or ventricular) beats are present as seen in this case.

It must be remembered that the term "A-V dissociation" is *not* a complete rhythm diagnosis because it is always due to some other basic cardiac rhythm disorder(s). Thus, the A-V dissociation is analogous to various clinical manifestations such as fever, anemia, or jaundice, which may be due to numerous underlying disorders.

Left ventricular hypertrophy can be diagnosed without any difficulty (see Case 10).

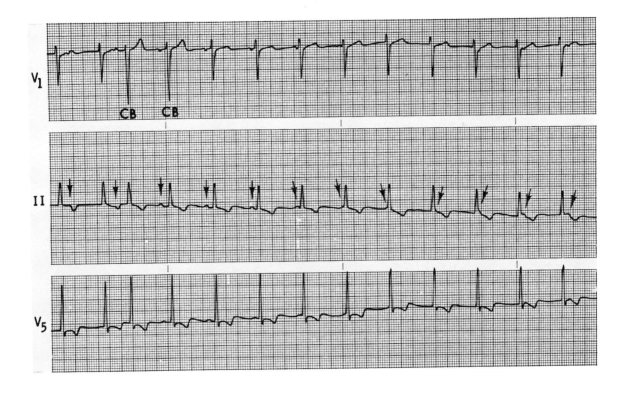

V₁

CB   CB

II

V₅

CASE 117

During digitalization, the cardiac rhythm is found to be regular in a 61-year-old man with chronic atrial fibrillation or flutter–fibrillation with congestive heart failure due to hypertensive heart disease.

1. *What is your cardiac rhythm diagnosis?*
2. *What is the most likely direct cause of this rhythm disorder?*
3. *What other ECG abnormality is present?*

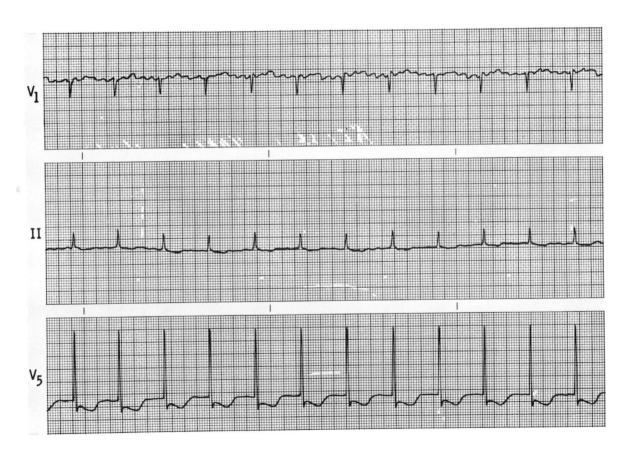

CASE 117: DIAGNOSIS

The underlying cardiac rhythm is atrial flutter–fibrillation, but the R-R interval is precisely regular. Thus, a complete cardiac rhythm diagnosis is atrial flutter–fibrillation with nonparoxysmal A-V junctional tachycardia (ventricular rate 83 beats per minute) producing complete A-V dissociation.

In this case, nonparoxysmal A-V junctional tachycardia is responsible for the production of complete A-V dissociation (see Case 116). The cause for the genesis of nonparoxysmal A-V junctional tachycardia is, needless to say, digitalis intoxication. It should be re-emphasized that the most common cause of nonparoxysmal A-V junctional tachycardia is digitalis intoxication.

It is easy to recognize the evidence of left ventricular hypertrophy. In addition, coarse atrial fibrillation or atrial flutter–fibrillation often suggests left atrial hypertrophy.

CASE 118

This ECG tracing was obtained from a 79-year-old woman with recent myocardial infarction associated with congestive heart failure. During rapid digitalization, her cardiac rhythm has been changed.

1. What is your cardiac rhythm diagnosis?
2. What is the other ECG abnormality?

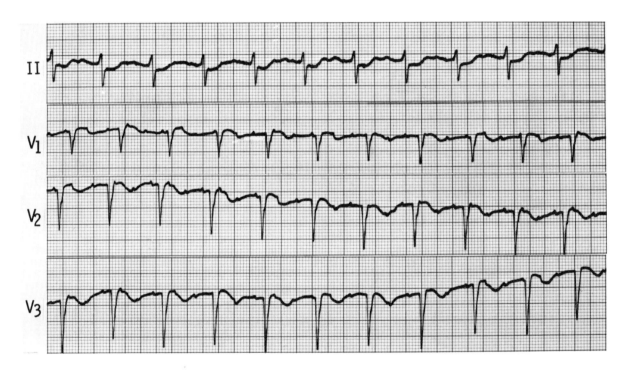

CASE 118: DIAGNOSIS

Arrows indicate P waves. The cardiac rhythm reveals atrial tachycardia (atrial rate 230 beats per minute, indicated by *arrows)* with nonparoxysmal A-V junctional tachycardia (ventricular rate 95 beats per minute) producing complete A-V dissociation. Note that there is no relationship between atrial and ventricular activities. Thus, the rhythm diagnosis is double supraventricular tachycardia causing complete A-V dissociation. This type of cardiac rhythm disorder is a characteristic feature of digitalis intoxication.

The diagnosis of recent anteroseptal myocardial infarction is obvious (Q-S waves in leads V_1 through V_3 with T wave inversion and S-T segment elevation; see Chapter 3), and marked left axis deviation of the QRS complexes (QRS axis −45°, calculated from a 12-lead ECG) represent left anterior hemiblock (see Chapter 10).

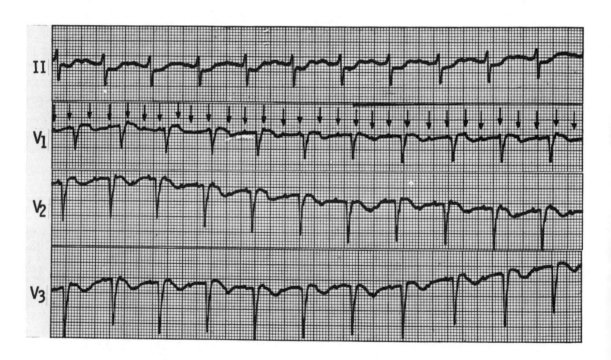

CASE 119

These cardiac rhythm strips were obtained from a 59-year-old man with chronic congestive heart failure associated with chronic atrial fibrillation due to hypertensive heart disease. Digitalis toxicity was suspected.

What is your cardiac rhythm diagnosis?

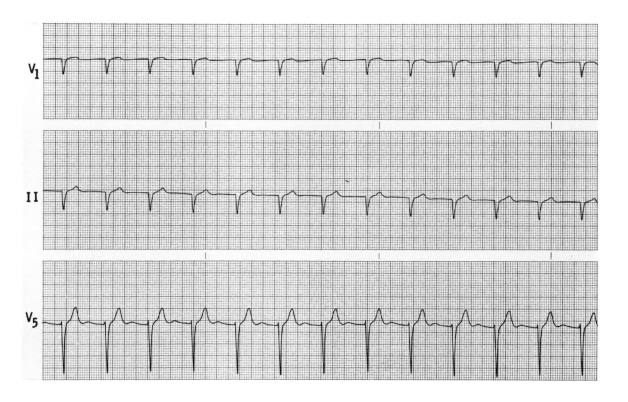

CASE 119: DIAGNOSIS

No clear atrial activity is discernible, but it is not uncommon in a fine fibrillation as seen in coronary and/or hypertensive heart disease. The cardiac rhythm is atrial fibrillation with nonparoxysmal A-V junctional tachycardia (ventricular rate 82 beats per minute) producing complete A-V dissociation. As repeatedly emphasized, nonparoxysmal A-V junctional tachycardia, especially in the presence of the pre-existing atrial fibrillation, is the most common arrhythmia in digitalis intoxication. Thus, digitalis toxicity should be immediately suspected in patients with atrial fibrillation when the cardiac rhythm is found to be regular during digitalization (either during rapid administration or during a maintenance digitalis therapy).

Left anterior hemiblock is diagnosed on the basis of marked left axis deviation of the QRS complexes (QRS axis −60°, calculated from a 12-lead ECG).

CASE 120

A 61-year-old man was admitted to the Coronary Care Unit because of severe chest pain of 8–10 hours' duration.

1. *What is your cardiac rhythm diagnosis?*
2. *What is the treatment of choice for this rhythm disorder?*

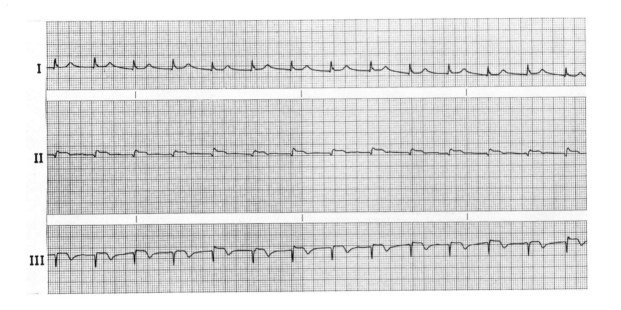

CASE 120: DIAGNOSIS

Arrows indicate sinus P waves. The cardiac rhythm discloses marked sinus bradycardia (indicated by *arrows,* atrial rate 38 beats per minute) with nonparoxysmal A-V junctional tachycardia (ventricular rate 84 beats per minute) producing complete A-V dissociation. Note that the atrial and ventricular activities are independent throughout the tracing. In this case, there are two factors responsible for A-V dissociation: marked sinus bradycardia and nonparoxysmal A-V junctional tachycardia (see Case 116).

The diagnosis of acute diaphragmatic (inferior) myocardial infarction can be made without any difficulty on the basis of pathologic (abnormal) Q waves in leads II, III, and aVF (not shown here).

It has been well documented that nonparoxysmal A-V junctional tachycardia is common in acute diaphragmatic myocardial infarction, particularly during the first 24–72 hours. This cardiac rhythm disorder is, as a rule, self-limited, and no treatment is indicated. Similarly, marked sinus bradycardia requires no treatment in this case, as long as the patient maintains an adequate ventricular rate.

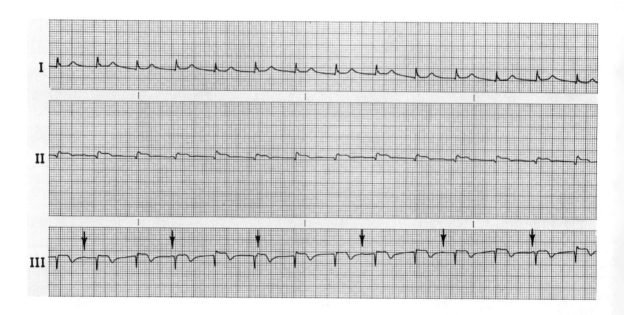

CASE 121

This ECG tracing was obtained postoperatively from a 55-year-old woman with aortic stenosis. Aortic valve replacement was performed.

What is your cardiac rhythm diagnosis?

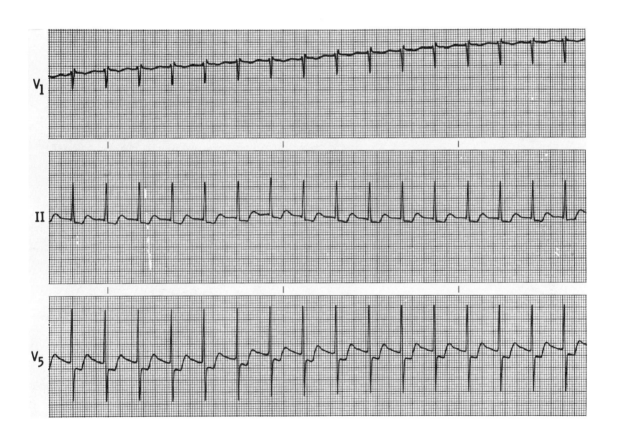

CASE 121: DIAGNOSIS

The cardiac rhythm is nonparoxysmal A-V junctional tachycardia with a rate of 108 beats per minute. No P waves are discernible. Thus, the rhythm is probably a pure A-V junctional tachycardia in that the P waves and the QRS complexes are superimposed leading to absence of inverted P waves. However, a fine atrial fibrillation cannot be entirely excluded.

Nonparoxysmal A-V junctional tachycardia, observed postoperatively, is usually self-limited, and the arrhythmia seldom lasts more than 3 days after surgery. Thus, no treatment is indicated for the arrhythmia.

Left ventricular hypertrophy is strongly suggested (see Case 10).

CASE 122

Digitalis intoxication was diagnosed in a 78-year-old woman with chronic atrial fibrillation and previous history of myocardial infarction 1 year ago.

1. *What is your cardiac rhythm diagnosis?*
2. *What other ECG abnormality is present?*

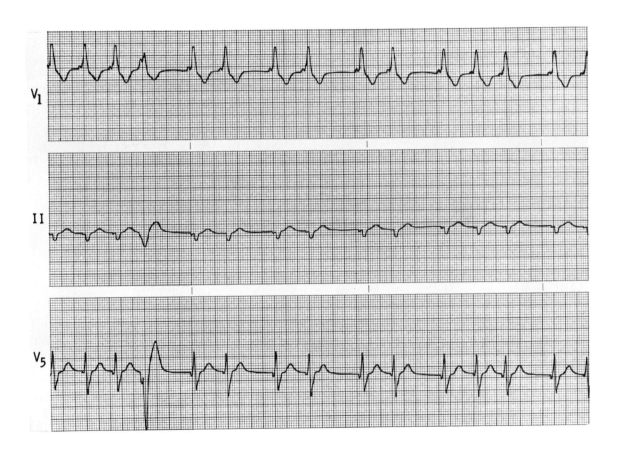

CASE 122: DIAGNOSIS

The cardiac rhythm appears to show frequent ventricular group beats followed by ventricular pauses. The ventricular group beats consist of predominantly two QRS complexes and intermittently three QRS complexes. In addition, the R-R intervals progressively shorten (more obvious in three grouped QRS complexes) until a ventricular pause occurs. Furthermore, the longest R-R interval (ventricular pause) is shorter than two of the shortest R-R intervals. This ECG finding is a characteristic feature of Wenckebach phenomenon (see Case 131).

Thus, a final rhythm diagnosis of this ECG tracing is a fine atrial fibrillation and nonparoxysmal A-V junctional tachycardia (rate 124 beats per minute) with predominantly 3:2 (occasionally 4:3) Wenckebach exit block producing complete A-V dissociation (see also Cases 116 and 131). Note a ventricular premature contraction (fourth QRS complex).

This cardiac rhythm disorder is a typical example of a far-advanced digitalis intoxication.

It is easy to recognize the evidence of right bundle branch block, but the QRS contour is *not* typical for a pure right bundle branch block. Namely, the QRS complex in lead V₁ is entirely above the isoelectric line which means a loss of posterior force—posterior myocardial infarction. Therefore, the diagnosis of diaphragmatic posterolateral myocardial infarction can be made (see Chapter 3, Case 48).

CASE 123

These cardiac rhythm strips were obtained from a 52-year-old man with coronary heart disease.

What is your cardiac rhythm diagnosis?

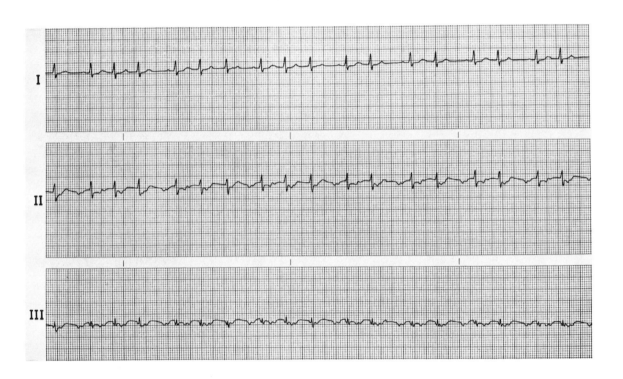

CASE 123: DIAGNOSIS

Arrows indicate retrograde P waves. The cardiac rhythm is paroxysmal A-V junctional tachycardia (indicated by *arrows;* atrial rate 162 beats per minute) with 3:2 (occasionally 4:3) Wenckebach A-V block (see Case 131). Note that a typical feature of a progressive shortening of the R-R intervals is *not* shown during 4:3 A-V conduction. Thus, the finding has to be called atypical Wenckebach A-V block which is not uncommon in our practice. Reciprocating (re-entrant) tachycardia with Wenckebach A-V block is an alternative rhythm diagnosis.

This patient had suffered from diaphragmatic myocardial infarction 3 weeks previously (Q waves in leads III and aVF, not shown here), and this type of rhythm disorder is somewhat unusual in diaphragmatic myocardial infarction. The arrhythmia has subsided spontaneously, and the patient was asymptomatic. Note a low voltage of the QRS complexes which is common in patients with myocardial infarction (see Case 32).

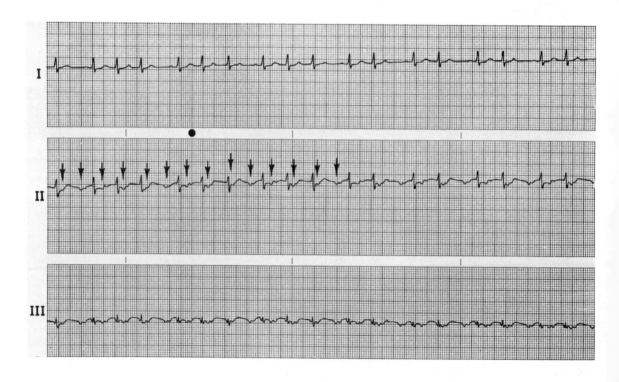

CASE 124

This ECG tracing was obtained from a 30-year-old woman with no demonstrable heart disease.

What is your cardiac rhythm diagnosis?

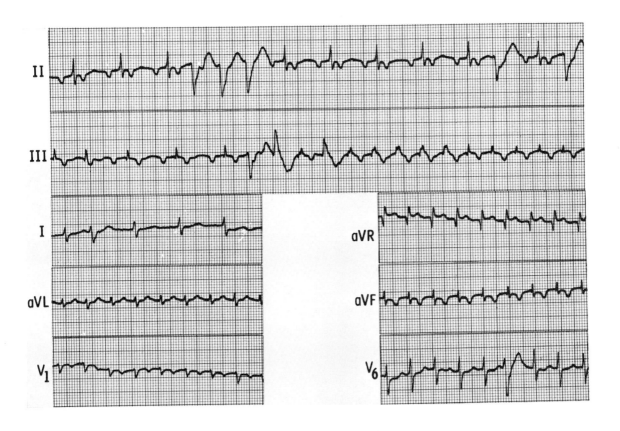

CASE 124: DIAGNOSIS

Arrows indicate retrograde P waves. The cardiac rhythm is reciprocating (re-entrant) tachycardia with 1:1 A-V conduction with intermittent varying Wenckebach A-V block and 2:1 A-V block. There are also frequent bizarre QRS complexes (marked X) due to aberrant ventricular conduction. The aberrantly conducted beats closely resemble ventricular premature contractions (marked X).

Reciprocating tachycardia is considered to be due to a re-entry phenomenon which occurs in the A-V junction as a result of uneven depression of the conductivity—longitudinal dissociation in the A-V junctional tissue.

Clinically, reciprocating tachycardia is *not* specific for any particular clinical circumstance. This rhythm disorder may be found in digitalis toxicity. However, this patient fails to show any evidence of heart disease, and, of course, she is not taking digitalis. Whenever dealing with young individuals complaining of any type of ectopic tachycardia, possible causes such as excessive use of coffee, tea, or Coca-Cola, heavy smoking, Wolff-Parkinson-White syndrome, and hyperthyroidism should always be considered. Otherwise, mitral valve prolapse syndrome, rheumatic heart disease, and any other organic heart diseases should be investigated.

No direct cause for the arrhythmia was found in this patient. The small oral dosage of propranolol (Inderal, 10 mg 4 times a day) was effective in eliminating her tachycardia. Therefore, her arrhythmia is considered to be catecholamine-induced.

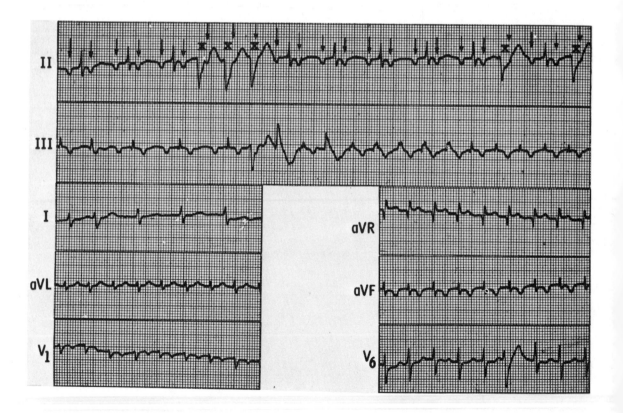

CASE 125

These cardiac rhythm strips were obtained from a 50-year-old woman with chronic congestive heart failure due to rheumatic heart disease. Digitalis intoxication was suspected.

What is your cardiac rhythm diagnosis?

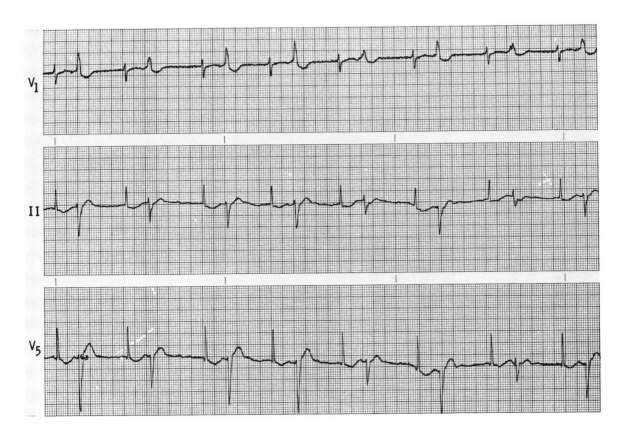

CASE 125: DIAGNOSIS

The underlying cardiac rhythm is atrial fibrillation, but the R-R intervals are regular in many areas. Thus, the basic rhythm is atrial fibrillation with frequent A-V junctional escape beats due to high degree (advanced) A-V block. In addition, there are frequent ventricular premature contractions producing ventricular bigeminy. This type of cardiac arrhythmia is almost a pathognomonic feature of digitalis toxicity.

Furthermore, ventricular premature contractions originating from the left ventricle seem to be much more common in digitalis intoxication than those arising from the right ventricle. It should be noted that left ventricular premature contractions reveal right bundle branch block pattern, and vice versa.

CASE 126

This ECG tracing was obtained from a 64-year-old woman with coronary heart disease following cardiac arrest.

1. *What is your cardiac rhythm diagnosis?*
2. *What other ECG abnormality is present?*

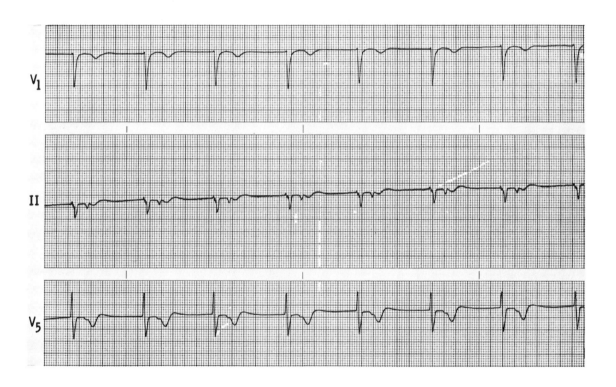

CASE 126: DIAGNOSIS

Arrows indicate retrograde P waves. The cardiac rhythm exhibits A-V junctional escape rhythm with a rate of 48 beats per minute. Note that each QRS complex is followed by a retrograde P wave (indicated by *arrows*) with prolonged R-P interval (R-P interval 0.24 second). The prolonged R-P interval indicates a delayed retrograde ventriculoatrial (V-A) conduction.

The T waves are inverted in practically all leads (only three leads are shown in this tracing) indicative of diffuse myocardial ischemia which is common immediately after cardiac arrest. The diffuse T wave change may also be due to central nervous system disorder (cerbral hypoxia due to cardiac arrest).

Another ECG abnormality is left anterior hemiblock (see Chapter 10).

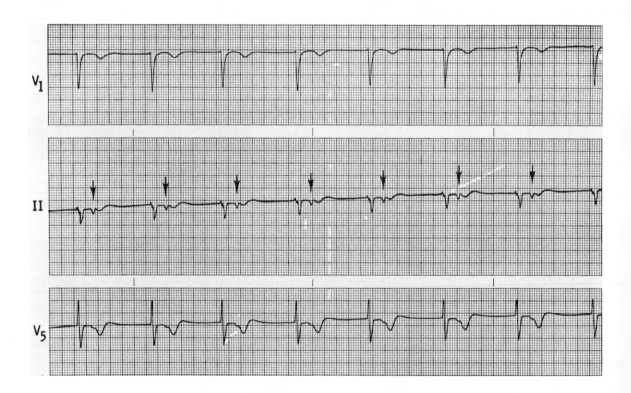

CASE 127

Digitalis intoxication was diagnosed in a 77-year-old man with hypertensive heart disease on the basis of marked slowing of the heart rate associated with worsening of congestive heart failure.

1. What is your cardiac rhythm diagnosis?
2. Is artificial pacing indicated?

CASE 127: DIAGNOSIS

The underlying cardiac rhythm is atrial fibrillation, but the ventricular cycle is regular with slow ventricular rate. Thus, the rhythm diagnosis is atrial fibrillation with A-V junctional escape rhythm (ventricular rate 45 beats per minute) due to complete A-V block resulting in complete A-V dissociation (see Chapter 8).

Under this circumstance, two major factors, ventricular rate and presence or absence of symptom (*e.g.,* fainting, dizziness, hypotension, etc.), will determine the indication or nonindication of the artificial pacing. In general, an artificial pacemaker is considered to be indicated when the ventricular rate in complete A-V block is slower than 45 beats per minute. An artificial pacemaker is definitely indicated for symptomatic complete A-V block. As a rule, the patient with complete A-V block is often symptomatic when the ventricular rate of the escape rhythm is slower than 45 beats per minute.

Needless to say, discontinuation of digitalis is the first and the most important therapeutic approach for the patient with digitalis intoxication.

Left ventricular hypertrophy is suspected, and prominent U waves are suggestive of hypokalemia. It is well documented that hypokalemia frequently predisposes to digitalis toxicity.

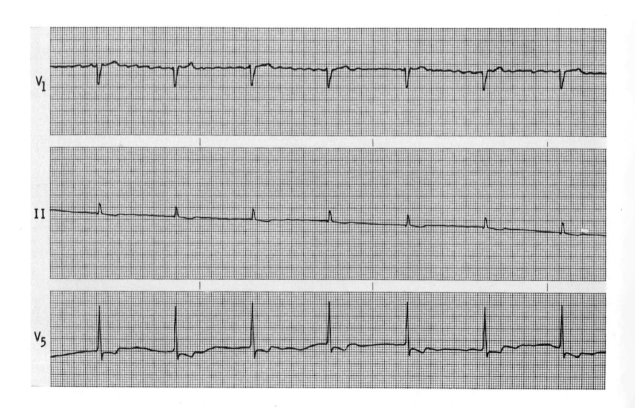

CASE 128

This electrocardiogram was obtained from a 72-year-old woman with mild hypertension.

What is your cardiac rhythm diagnosis?

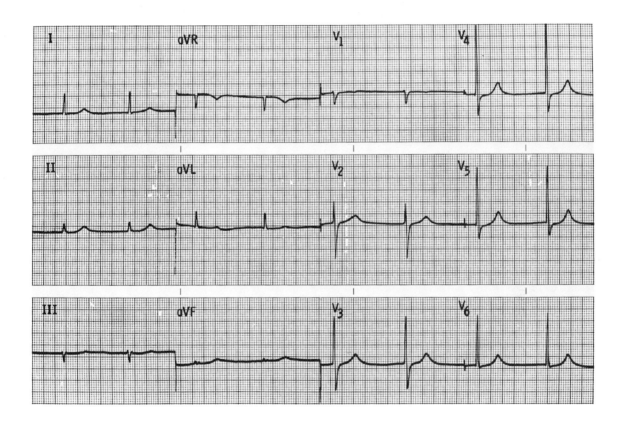

CASE 128: DIAGNOSIS

No P waves are discernible, but the ventricular cycle is regular with normal QRS complexes. Thus, the cardiac rhythm reveals A-V junctional escape rhythm with a rate of 48 beats per minute. In this tracing, the atrial mechanism may be a fine atrial fibrillation, so that the rhythm diagnosis may be atrial fibrillation with A-V junctional escape rhythm due to complete A-V block resulting in complete A-V dissociation. On the other hand, the A-V junctional pacemaker may activate the atria and the ventricles simultaneously, leading to absence of retrograde P waves because of their superimposition to the QRS complexes. It is impossible to distinguish these two possibilities from the surface electrocardiogram.

Left ventricular hypertrophy is suggested primarily from the voltage criteria (see Case 10).

CASE 129

Digitalis intoxication was suspected in a 68-year-old man with a permanent artificial (ventricular) pacemaker.

What is your cardiac rhythm diagnosis?

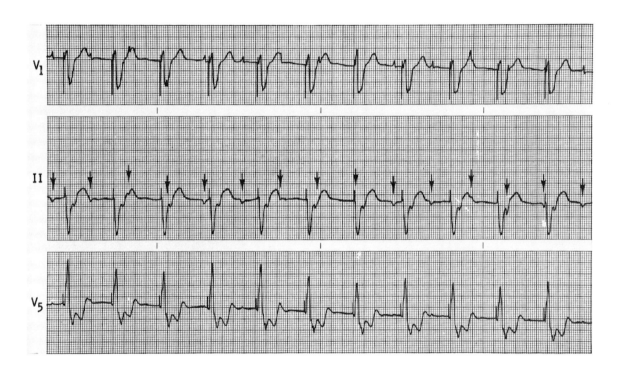

CASE 129: DIAGNOSIS

Arrows indicate retrograde P waves. It is easy to recognize an artificial pacemaker-induced ventricular rhythm with a rate of 67 beats per minute. By close observation, regularly occurring retrograde P waves (inverted P waves in lead II) with a rate of 85 beats per minute can be appreciated. Thus, a complete cardiac rhythm diagnosis is nonparoxysmal A-V junctional tachycardia (atrial rate 85 beats per minute) with an artificial pacemaker-induced ventricular rhythm (ventricular rate 67 beats per minute) producing complete A-V dissociation.

It should be emphasized that patients with artificial pacemakers are *not* immune to digitalis toxicity. The recognition of the alteration in the atrial mechanism, particularly the development of nonparoxysmal A-V junctional tachycardia or atrial tachycardia, in the presence of an artificial pacemaker-induced ventricular rhythm is often a key factor in the diagnosis of digitalis toxicity. In addition, frequent ventricular premature contractions in the presence of an artificial pacemaker rhythm often indicate digitalis toxicity.

chapter 8

ATRIOVENTRICULAR (A-V) CONDUCTION DISTURBANCES

CASE 130

The ECG tracing shown on this page was taken on admission (tracing A), whereas another ECG tracing shown on the next page (tracing B) was recorded 3 days after discontinuation of digitalis. Digitalis intoxication was diagnosed in an 84-year-old man with hypertensive heart disease.

What is your cardiac rhythm diagnosis?

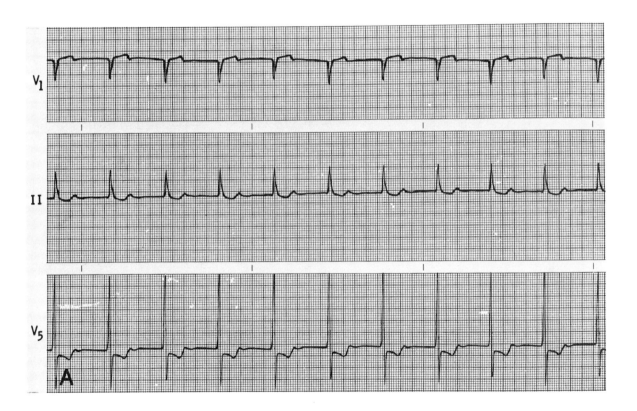

CASE 130: DIAGNOSIS

The cardiac rhythm of the tracing A appears to be A-V junctional escape rhythm because no P waves are clearly visible. A false impression of absent P waves is simply due to the fact that all P waves are superimposed on the top of the T waves of the preceding beats. Accordingly, the cardiac rhythm in tracing A is sinus rhythm with marked first degree A-V block (P-R interval 0.62 second).

The P-R intervals become markedly shortened on discontinuation of digitalis within 3 days as shown in tracing B. In tracing B, first degree A-V block is still present, but the P-R interval is only 0.30 second.

The diagnosis of left atrial as well as left ventricular hypertrophy can be made without any difficulty (see Cases 10 and 11).

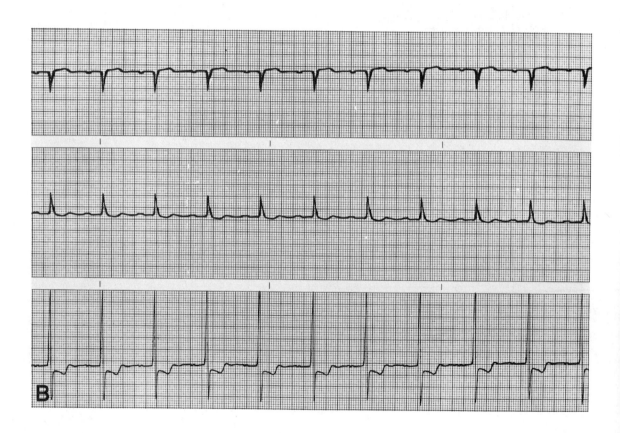

CASE 131

These cardiac rhythm strips were obtained from a 75-year-old man with chronic congestive heart failure due to hypertensive heart disease. Digitalis intoxication was suspected.

What is your cardiac rhythm diagnosis?

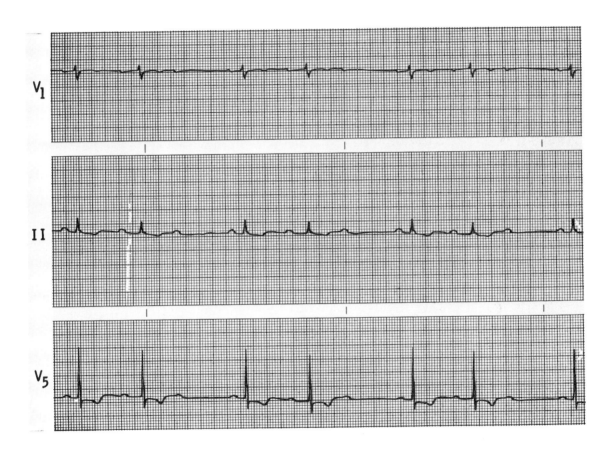

CASE 131: DIAGNOSIS

The cardiac rhythm reveals sinus rhythm (atrial rate 72 beats per minute) with 3:2 Wenckebach (Mobitz type-I) A-V block. Note a progressive lengthening of the P-R intervals followed by a blocked P wave. The term "3:2 A-V block" is used when every third P wave is not conducted to the ventricles. In other words, two out of three P waves are conducted to the ventricles. In Wenckebach A-V block, the ventricular cycles (R-R intervals) are progressively shortened until a ventricular pause occurs. When the A-V conduction ratio is 3:2, short and long R-R intervals alternate leading to a ventricular pseudo-bigeminy. The long R-R interval is shorter than two P-P cycles.

The fundamental mechanism responsible for Wenckebach A-V block is diagrammatically illustrated in this page. The numbers represent hundredths of a second. The numbers in the upper row represent the atrial cycle (P-P interval) with a rate of 60 beats per minute. The numbers within the oblique lines at the A-V level indicate the A-V conduction time (P-R interval). The progressive lengthening of the P-R intervals is apparent until a blocked atrial impulse (dropped P wave) occurs. Following this blocked atrial impulse, the P-R interval shortens to its original value (0.20 second), and the sequence is repeated. The numbers in the lower row represent the duration of successive ventricular cycles. The progressive shortening of the ventricular cycle length (R-R interval) is due to the progressive increment of A-V conduction before the blocked atrial impulse and the decrement immediately following the blocked P wave. The numbers in parentheses in the lower row indicate the degree of increment or decrement in the ventricular cycle length.

Wenckebach (Mobitz type-I) A-V block is very common in digitalis intoxication, while Mobitz type-II A-V block (Case 136) has not been reported as a manifestation of digitalis toxicity.

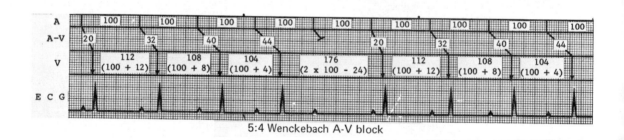

5:4 Wenckebach A-V block

CASE 132

A 48-year-old woman was admitted to the Coronary Care Unit because of severe chest pain of 5–6 hours' duration.

1. *What is your cardiac rhythm diagnosis?*
2. *What is the other ECG abnormality?*
3. *What is the treatment of choice for this rhythm disorder?*

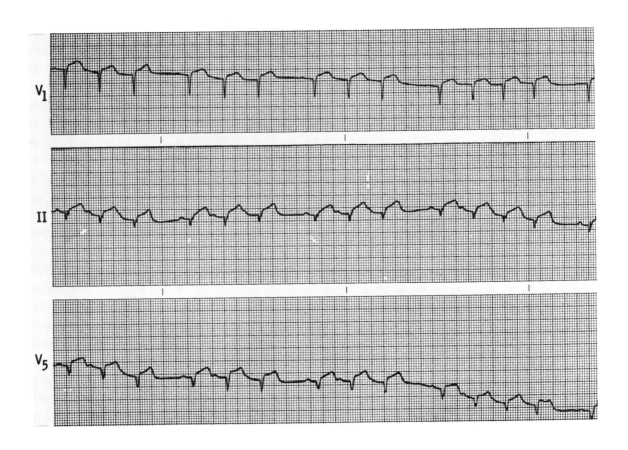

CASE 132: DIAGNOSIS

Arrows indicate sinus P waves. The cardiac rhythm reveals sinus tachycardia (indicated by *arrows;* atrial rate 120 beats per minute) with 4:3 and intermittent 5:4 Wenckebach A-V block. Note a progressive lengthening of the P-R intervals until a ventricular pause occurs. Detailed descriptions of Wenckebach A-V block can be found elsewhere (see Case 131).

Acute diaphragmatic (inferior)—lateral myocardial infarction is readily diagnosed on the basis of Q or Q-S waves with S-T segment elevation in leads II, III, aVF, and V_4 through V_6 (only leads II and V_5 are shown here).

Wenckebach A-V block is extremely common during the first 24–72 hours of acute diaphragmatic myocardial infarction as a result of impairment of blood supply to the A-V junction. Wenckebach A-V block is self-limited in most cases with acute diaphragmatic myocardial infarction, and no treatment is necessary as long as the arrhythmia is asymptomatic.

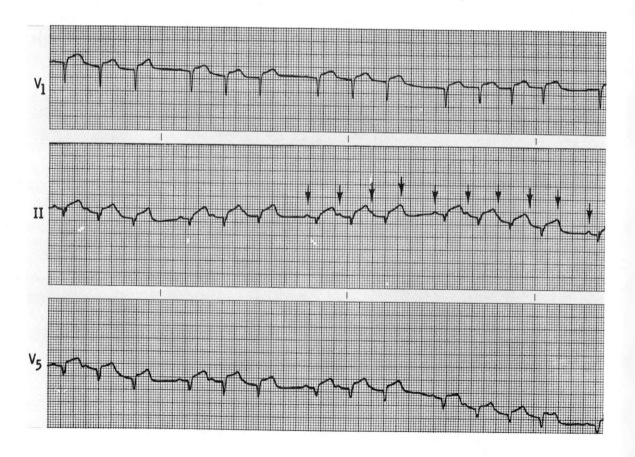

CASE 133

A 77-year-old man was admitted to the Coronary Care Unit because of severe chest pain of 12 hours' duration.

     1. What is your cardiac rhythm diagnosis?
     2. What is the other ECG abnormality?
     3. What is the treatment of choice for this rhythm disorder?

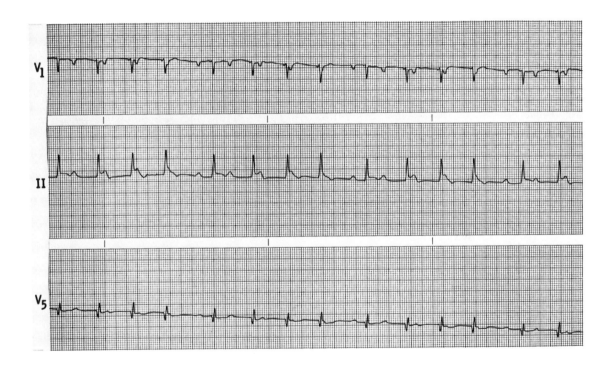

CASE 133: DIAGNOSIS

Arrows indicate sinus P waves. The cardiac rhythm discloses sinus tachycardia (indicated by *arrows;* atrial rate 108 beats per minute) with varying (5:4 and 4:3) Wenckebach (Mobitz type-I) A-V block. It should be noted that many P waves are partially or even totally superimposed on the QRS complexes of the preceding beats, leading to a false appearance of absent P waves in some areas. This occurs primarily because of a slowly progressing Wenckebach A-V block in addition to a relatively rapid sinus rate. By close observation, however, three or four grouped QRS complexes followed by a ventricular pause are readily recognized. In addition, a progressive lengthening of the P-R intervals with a concomitant progressive shortening of the R-R intervals (ventricular cycles) can be appreciated before a blocked P wave occurs. These ECG findings are, of course, the characteristic features of Wenckebach (Mobitz type-I) A-V block (see Case 131).

This patient has suffered from acute diaphragmatic and extensive anterior myocardial infarction (only three leads are shown here). The direct underlying cause for the development of Wenckebach A-V block is considered to be acute diaphragmatic myocardial infarction as a result of impairment of blood supply to the A-V junction. The reason for this is that, in the majority of cases, diaphragmatic myocardial infarction occurs as a result of right coronary artery occlusion, and the blood vessel supplying the A-V junction primarily branches off the right coronary artery in most cases. Thus, acute ischemic changes in the A-V junction are considered to be responsible for the production of Wenckebach A-V block (see Cases 132–134) as well as nonparoxysmal A-V junctional tachycardia (see Case 120) in acute diaphragmatic myocardial infarction.

As mentioned previously, Wenckebach A-V block associated with acute diaphragmatic myocardial infarction is self-limited in nearly all cases. Thus, no treatment is indicated under this circumstance as long as the ideal ventricular rate (ventricular rate faster than 50 beats per minute) is maintained.

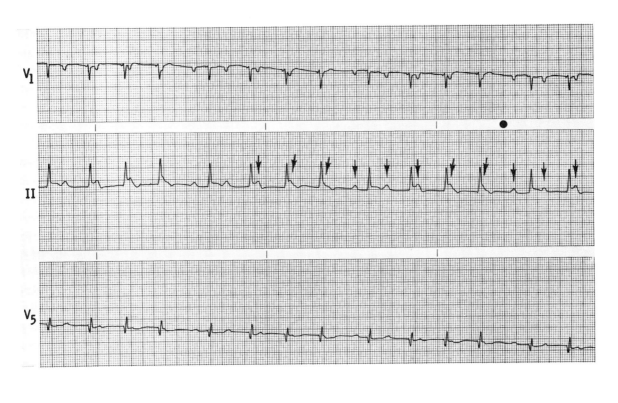

CASE 134

These cardiac rhythm strips were obtained from a 74-year-old woman with recent myocardial infarction. Her slow heart rate was found to be asymptomatic.

1. What is your cardiac rhythm diagnosis?
2. What is the treatment of choice?

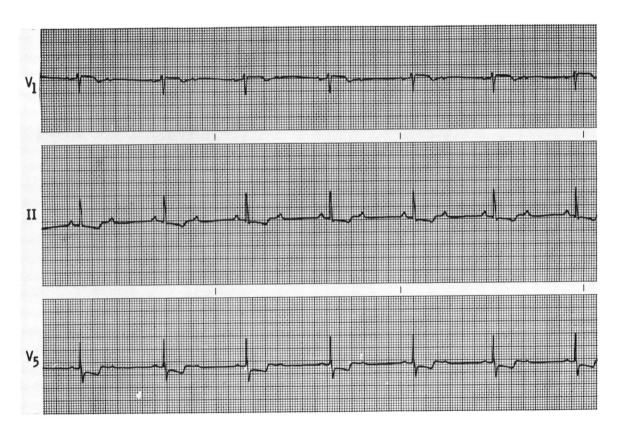

CASE 134: DIAGNOSIS

Arrows indicate sinus P waves. The cardiac rhythm reveals sinus rhythm (indicated by *arrows;* atrial rate 90 beats per minute) with 2:1 A-V block. Note that every other P wave is not conducted to the ventricles.

The diagnosis of recent diaphragmatic myocardial infarction was made on the basis of abnormal Q waves in leads III and aVF (not shown here) associated with S-T, T wave changes.

When dealing with 2:1 A-V block, the type of A-V block cannot be determined with a certainty unless there is a transitional change from or to Mobitz type-I or -II A-V block on the same ECG tracing. Nevertheless, a variant of Wenckebach (Mobitz type-I) A-V block is almost certain when the QRS complex is normal in configuration in 2:1 A-V block. This is particularly true in patients with recent diaphragmatic myocardial infarction or digitalis intoxication.

As far as the management is concerned, no treatment is necessary for asymptomatic 2:1 A-V block which is a variant of Wenckebach A-V block in recent diaphragmatic myocardial infarction as long as the ventricular rate is faster than 45 beats per minute. However, the patient should be observed closely for a possible development of complete A-V block with slower ventricular rate.

There is a significant controversy regarding the use of an artificial pacemaker in acute myocardial infarction. In general, an artificial pacemaker is considered to be definitely indicated for *symptomatic* bradyarrhythmias (including marked sinus bradycardia, second degree and complete A-V block). The prophylactic pacing is recommended for a bifascicular or trifascicular block (see Cases 164 and 166) with acute onset in patients with acute myocardial infarction. Occasionally, overdriving pacing is a life-saving measure for refractory tachyarrhythmias, particularly ventricular tachycardia in acute myocardial infarction. However, the value of prophylactic pacing for hemiblocks or right bundle branch block alone (see Cases 156 and 162) due to acute myocardial infarction is not evident.

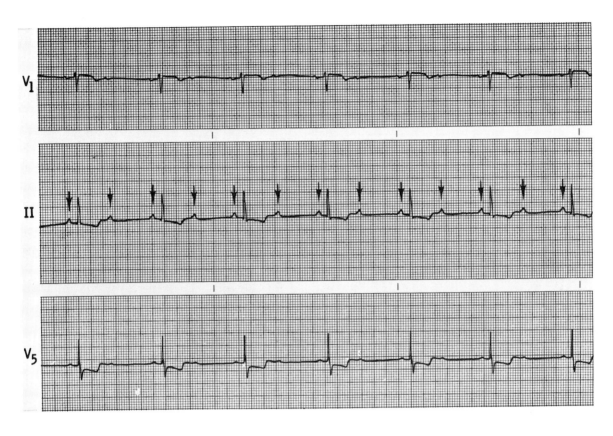

CASE 135

A 69-year-old man who had suffered from myocardial infarction 3 months previously was admitted to the Intermediate Coronary Care Unit because of fainting episodes. He was not taking any drug.

1. *What is your cardiac rhythm diagnosis?*
2. *What is the treatment of choice?*

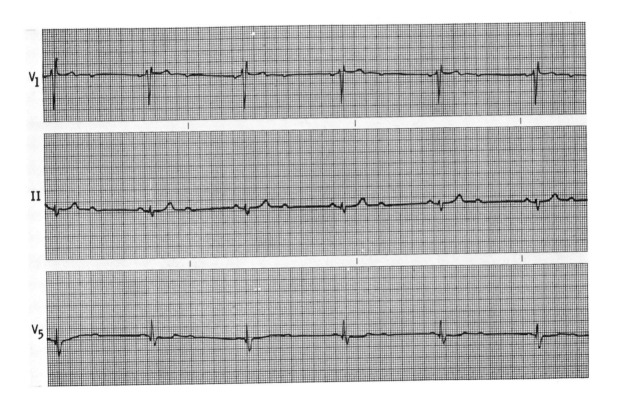

CASE 135: DIAGNOSIS

Arrows indicate sinus P waves. The cardiac rhythm exhibits sinus rhythm (indicated by *arrows;* atrial rate 70 beats per miunte) with 2:1 A-V block (ventricular rate 35 beats per minute). Note that every other P wave is conducted to the ventricles, and all conducted beats have constant P-R intervals.

Other ECG abnormalities include right bundle branch block and old diaphragmatic-lateral myocardial infarction (abnormal Q waves in leads II, III, aVF, and V_4 through V_6—only 3 leads are shown here).

When 2:1 A-V block is associated with right or left bundle branch block, or a bifascicular or trifascicular block, it is usually a variant of Mobitz type-II A-V block (see Cases 136 and 167) which is considered to be a precursor of complete A-V block due to complete trifascicular block (see Case 144). Thus, the site of the block under this circumstance is in the infranodal region.

As described previously, symptomatic A-V block requires an artificial pacemaker. This is particularly true in Mobitz type-II A-V block including 2:1 A-V block as a manifestation of Mobitz type-II A-V block, and complete A-V block due to complete trifascicular block. A permanent artificial pacemaker is indicated for chronic symptomatic second degree or complete A-V block. In second degree or complete A-V block, the ventricular rate slower than 45, particularly below 40, beats per minute usually produces significant symptoms for which artificial pacing is required.

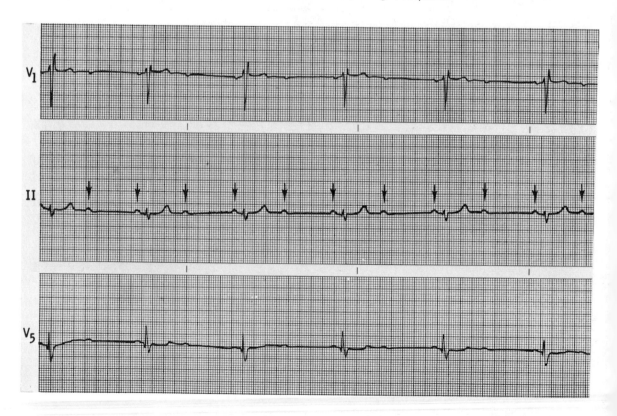

CASE 136

This electrocardiogram was obtained from a 72-year-old woman who has been suffering from lightheadedness. Myocardial infarction had occurred 6 months ago in this patient, but her recovery was uneventful. She was not taking any drug.

1. *What is your cardiac rhythm diagnosis?*
2. *Is artificial pacing indicated?*

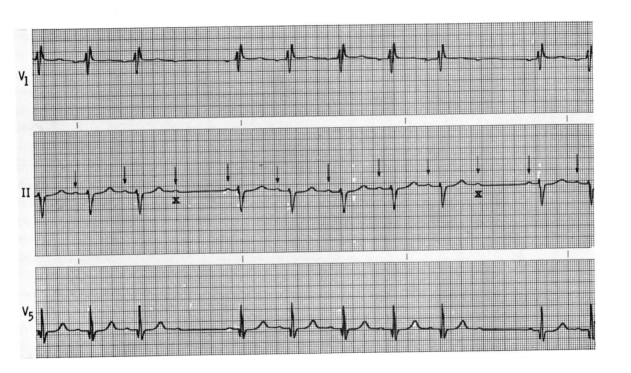

CASE 136: DIAGNOSIS

Arrows indicate sinus P waves. The cardiac rhythm reveals sinus rhythm (indicated by *arrows;* atrial rate 64 beats per minute) with first degree A-V block (P-R interval 0.24 second) and intermittent Mobitz type-II A-V block. Note that the P-R intervals remain constant in all conducted beats until a blocked P (marked *X*) occurs. Thus, the long P-R interval (ventricular pause) which contains a blocked P wave (marked *X*) is exactly two times the basic P-P cycles. These ECG findings are characteristic features of Mobitz type-II A-V block which represents infranodal block. It is well documented that Mobitz type-II A-V block is a precursor of complete A-V block due to complete trifascicular block (see Case 144).

In Mobitz type-II A-V block, the QRS complexes almost always demonstrate left or right bundle branch block or a bifascicular block (see Chapter 10). In this case, a combination of first degree A-V block with intermittent Mobitz type-II A-V block and a bifascicular block (right bundle branch block plus left anterior hemiblock) represents incomplete trifascicular block (incomplete bilateral bundle branch block; see Chapter 10).

This patient had suffered from extensive anterior myocardial infarction (except septum) 6 months ago, and abnormal Q waves are present in leads V_2 through V_6—only 3 leads are shown here).

She underwent permanent artificial pacemaker (demand unit) implantation. No further episode of lightheadedness was observed thereafter.

CASE 137

The ECG tracing shown on this page (tracing A) and another ECG tracing shown on the next page (tracing B) were obtained from an 82-year-old man with previous history of myocardial infarction 6 weeks ago. Tracings A and B were taken on the same day a few minutes apart.

What are your cardiac rhythm diagnoses of tracings A and B?

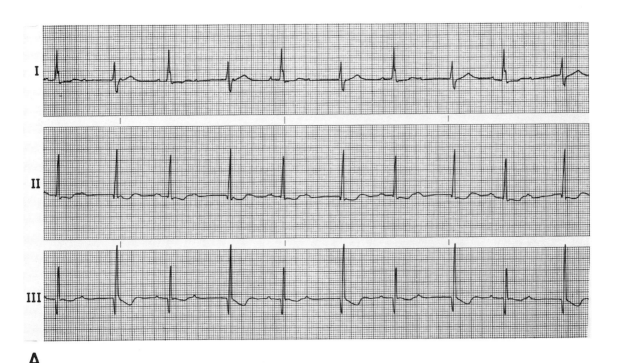

A

CASE 137: DIAGNOSIS

In tracing A, the basic rhythm is sinus rhythm (atrial rate 90 beats per minute) with 3:1 A-V block. There are frequent ventricular escape beats which alternate with basic sinus beats causing a form of ventricular bigeminy. When the escape beats alternate with the QRS complexes of the underlying rhythm (usually sinus rhythm), the term "ventricular escape-bigeminy" is used.

When dealing with 3:1 A-V block, again the type of A-V block cannot be determined with certainty unless a transitional change from or to Mobitz type-I or -II A-V block is found in the same ECG tracing. Otherwise, the type of A-V block can be judged from the finding of another ECG tracing obtained from the same individual as seen in this case.

That is, the cardiac rhythm shown in tracing B taken a few minutes later demonstrates sinus rhythm (indicated by *arrow;* atrial rate 90 beats per minute) with Wenckebach (Mobitz type-I) A-V block and frequent ventricular escape beats. Thus, the 3:1 A-V block in this patient is found to be a variant of Wenckebach A-V block. As repeatedly emphasized, a variant of Wenckebach A-V block is the most likely diagnosis when the QRS complexes of the conducted beats are normal in configuration in 2:1 or 3:1 A-V block.

Late development of A-V block (6 weeks following acute diaphragmatic myocardial infarction) is unusual following an acute coronary event. Therefore, the development of A-V block and myocardial infarction may not be directly related in this patient.

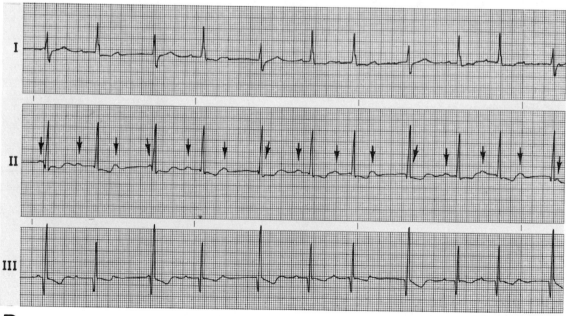

B

CASE 138

Digitalis intoxication was suspected in a 54-year-old man with rheumatic heart disease during a maintenance digitalis therapy because of extremely slow heart rate associated with aggravation of congestive heart failure. He was admitted to the Intermediate Coronary Care Unit for further evaluation and management.

1. What is your cardiac rhythm diagnosis?
2. Is artificial pacing indicated?

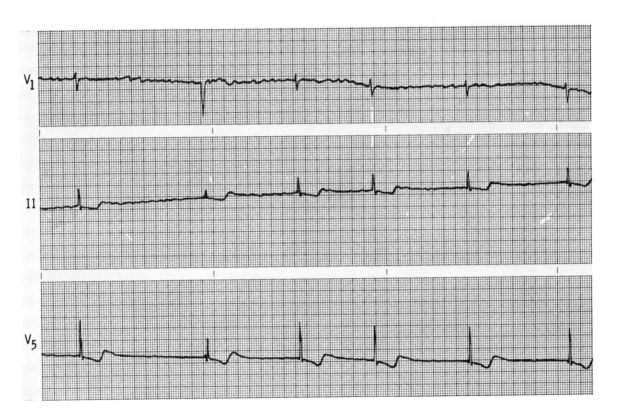

CASE 138: DIAGNOSIS

The underlying cardiac rhythm is coarse atrial fibrillation, but the ventricular rate is extremely slow (ventricular rate 30–40 beats per minute). When the ventricular rate is significantly slow (rate below 60 beats per minute), high-degree (advanced) A-V block is considered to be present in atrial fibrillation. When there is advanced A-V block in atrial fibrillation, the R-R intervals may be regular in some areas, but they may be grossly irregular. Regular and slow ventricular cycles with normal QRS complexes in atrial fibrillation indicate the presence of A-V junctional escape rhythm. Complete A-V block is diagnosed when the ventricular cycles are regular and slow (slower than 60 beats per minute) in atrial fibrillation (see Case 143).

In advanced A-V block, one or more ventricular escape beats may appear in atrial fibrillation. In this case, the escape beats are bizarre in configuration, and the escape interval is very long (the second beat in this tracing).

There are diffuse S-T, T wave changes which may represent digitalis effect. Coarse atrial fibrillation is indicative of left atrial hypertrophy (see Case 11).

When the ventricular rate is slower than 45 beats per minute, or advanced A-V block produces significant symptoms as seen in this patient, an artificial pacemaker is indicated. In most cases with digitalis-induced A-V block, temporary artificial pacing is sufficient in addition to discontinuation of digitalis.

CASE 139

These cardiac rhythm strips were obtained from a 76-year-old woman with recent myocardial infarction. There is no history of fainting episodes or dizziness.

1. *What is your cardiac rhythm diagnosis?*
2. *Is artificial pacing indicated?*

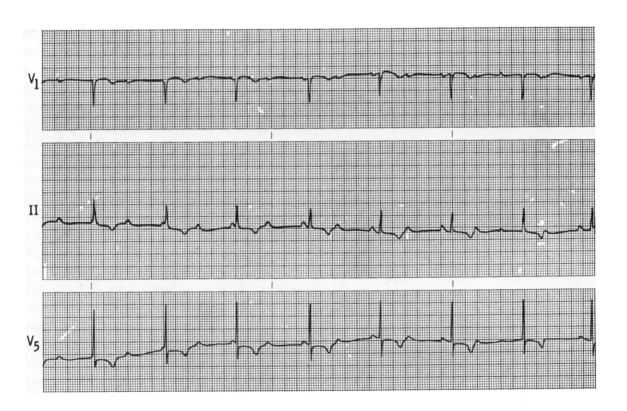

CASE 139: DIAGNOSIS

Arrows indicate sinus P waves. The cardiac rhythm reveals sinus tachycardia (indicated by *arrows;* atrial rate 105 beats per minute) with A-V junctional escape rhythm (ventricular rate 52 beats per minute) due to complete A-V block resulting in complete A-V dissociation. In addition, there is an atrial premature contraction (marked *A*).

The diagnosis of recent diaphragmatic myocardial infarction with diffuse anterior myocardial ischemia was made from a 12-lead ECG (not shown here).

Although significant controversy exists among physicians regarding the use of an artificial pacemaker in acute myocardial infarction, the artificial pacemaker is considered to be *not* indicated for asymptomatic complete A-V block, especially when the ventricular rate of the A-V junctional escape rhythm is above 50 beats per minute.

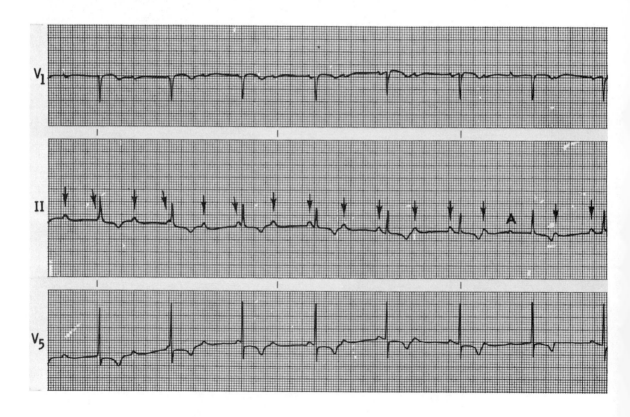

CASE 140

A 56-year-old man was admitted to the Coronary Care Unit because of severe chest pain associated with slow heart rate. He was hypotensive, and his mental status was slightly clouded on admission.

1. What is your cardiac rhythm diagnosis?
2. Is artificial pacing indicated?

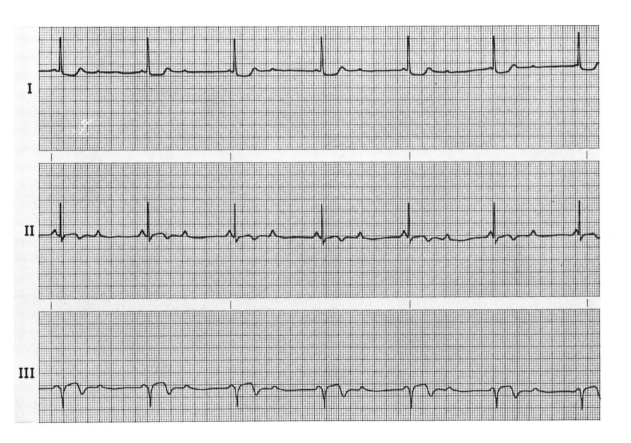

CASE 140: DIAGNOSIS

Arrows indicate sinus P waves. The cardiac rhythm reveals sinus rhythm (indicated by *arrows;* atrial rate 82 beats per minute) with A-V junctional escape rhythm (ventricular rate 42 beats per minute) due to complete A-V block resulting in complete A-V dissociation. The rhythm disorder superficially appears to be sinus rhythm with 2:1 A-V block. However, by close observation, it becomes obvious that the atrial and ventricular activities are independent throughout.

The site of complete A-V block in acute diaphragmatic myocardial infarction is intranodal block in which the escape pacemaker is located in the A-V junction. Thus, the QRS complexes of the escape rhythm demonstrate a normal (narrow) configuration in this case.

As repeatedly emphasized, symptomatic complete A-V block, especially when the ventricular rate is slower than 45 beats per minute, requires active treatment. Temporary artificial pacing is usually sufficient for symptomatic complete A-V block in acute diaphragmatic myocardial infarction because the A-V block, as a rule, is transient in most cases under this circumstance.

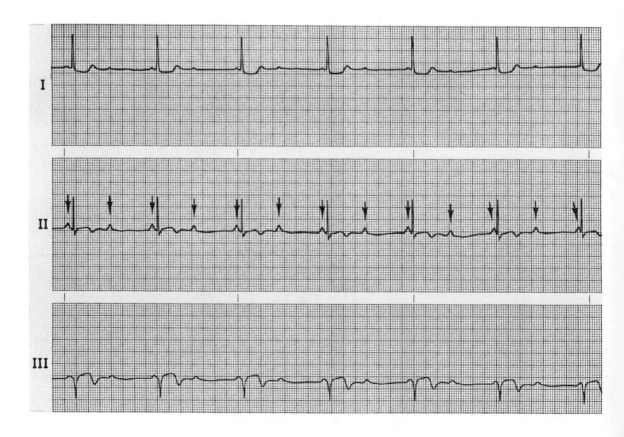

CASE 141

This electrocardiogram was obtained from a 24-year-old woman after surgical repair of a congenital heart disease. By reviewing tracings taken before surgery, the QRS complexes have been essentially unchanged postoperatively. The cardiac rhythm disorder shown on this ECG tracing has subsided within 48 hours after operation, and normal sinus rhythm was restored spontaneously. There was no history of fainting episodes as a result of this postoperative arrhythmia.

1. What is your cardiac rhythm diagnosis?
2. What is the underlying congenital cardiac defect?

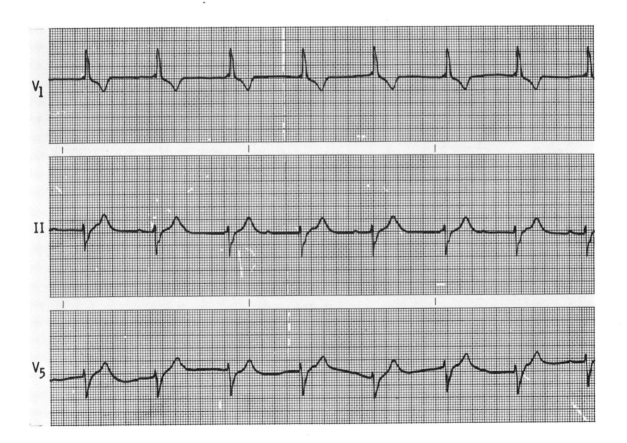

CASE 141: DIAGNOSIS

Arrows indicate sinus P waves. The cardiac rhythm shows sinus rhythm (indicated by *arrows;* atrial rate 88 beats per minute) with A-V junctional escape rhythm (ventricular rate 52 beats per minute) due to complete A-V block resulting in complete A-V dissociation.

As far as the configuration of the QRS complex is concerned, there is a combination of right bundle branch block and left anterior hemiblock (QRS axis −60°, calculated from a 12-lead ECG). Thus, a bifascicular block can be diagnosed (see Chapter 10). Among numerous congenital heart diseases, a bifascicular block consisting of right bundle branch block and left anterior hemiblock is nearly always found in patients with atrial septal defect, ostium primum type. Under this circumstance, a bifascicular block is considered to be congenital in origin.

Postoperative complete A-V block is often transient, and a restoration of sinus rhythm is observed spontaneously within 24–48 hours to 1 week after surgery. In this case, a transient inflammatory process in the A-V junction due to surgical trauma is considered to be responsible for the production of postoperative complete A-V block. On the other hand, a destructive surgical trauma to the conduction system, of course, may result in a permanent complete A-V block for which permanent artificial pacemaker implantation is indicated.

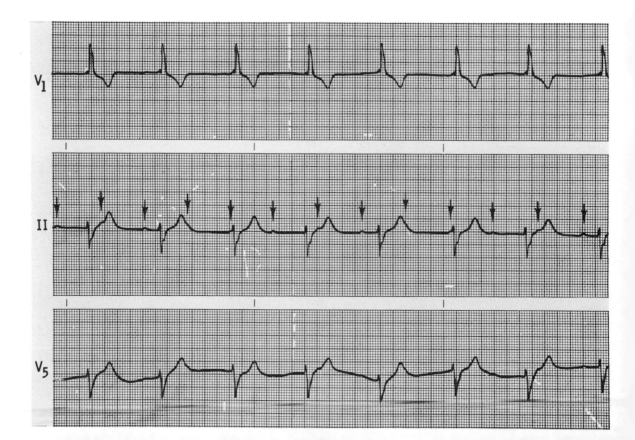

CASE 142

This electrocardiogram was obtained from a 59-year-old man with chronic congestive heart failure due to hypertensive heart disease. Digitalis intoxication was suspected.

1. *What is your cardiac rhythm diagnosis?*
2. *What is the treatment of choice?*

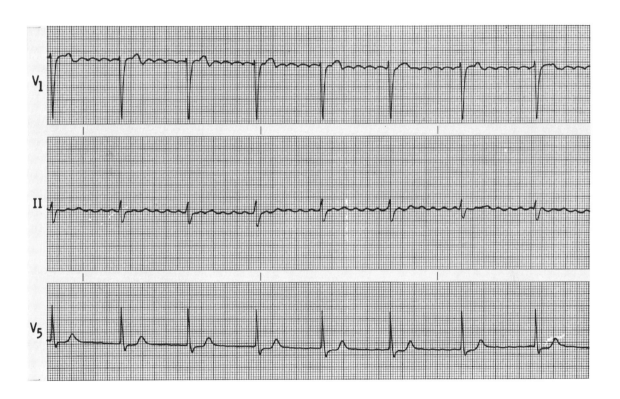

CASE 142: DIAGNOSIS

The cardiac rhythm is atrial flutter (atrial rate 320 beats per minute) with A-V junctional escape rhythm (ventricular rate 52 beats per minute) due to complete A-V block resulting in complete A-V dissociation. Note that the F-R intervals vary throughout, but the R-R intervals (ventricular cycles) remain constant with slow ventricular rate.

As emphasized previously, complete A-V block is most likely present when the A-V conduction ratio in atrial flutter appears to be more than 4:1. In complete A-V block, the atrial mechanism is not necessarily sinus rhythm. That is, the atrial mechanism in complete A-V block may be any ectopic rhythm such as atrial fibrillation, flutter, or tachycardia, and even A-V junctional tachycardia (see also Cases 127 and 143).

In digitalis-induced complete A-V block, the ventricular rate is reasonably well maintained (ventricular rate 45–60 beats per minute) because the escape rhythm is usually originating from the A-V junction. Therefore, complete A-V block *per se* in digitalis intoxication seldom produces significant symptoms such as fainting episodes. Accordingly, no active treatment such as artificial pacing is necessary other than discontinuation of digitalis.

Left ventricular hypertrophy is suggested (see Case 10).

CASE 143

Diagnosis of digitails toxicity was made on a 70-year-old man with chronic atrial fibrillation associated with chronic congestive heart failure due to hypertensive heart disease, because he developed markedly slow heart rate associated with aggravation of congestive heart failure.

1. *What is your cardiac rhythm diagnosis?*
2. *Is artificial pacing indicated?*

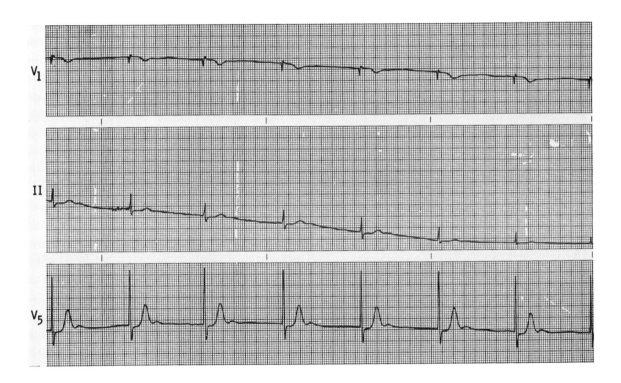

CASE 143: DIAGNOSIS

The cardiac rhythm is atrial fibrillation with A-V junctional escape rhythm (ventricular rate 43 beats per minute) due to complete A-V block resulting in complete A-V dissociation. Atrial activity is not clearly discernible because of a fine atrial fibrillation.

The use of temporary artificial pacing is considered to be definitely beneficial when the ventricular rate is slower than 45 beats per minute and/or the patient is symptomatic from complete A-V block itself as seen in this case. Of course, it is essential to discontinue digitalis immediately when digitalis intoxication is diagnosed.

Left ventricular hypertrophy is suggested (see Case 10).

CASE 144

An 80-year-old man was admitted to the Intermediate Coronary Care Unit because of Adams-Stokes syndrome. He was not taking any drug.

1. What is your cardiac rhythm diagnosis?
2. What is the treatment of choice?

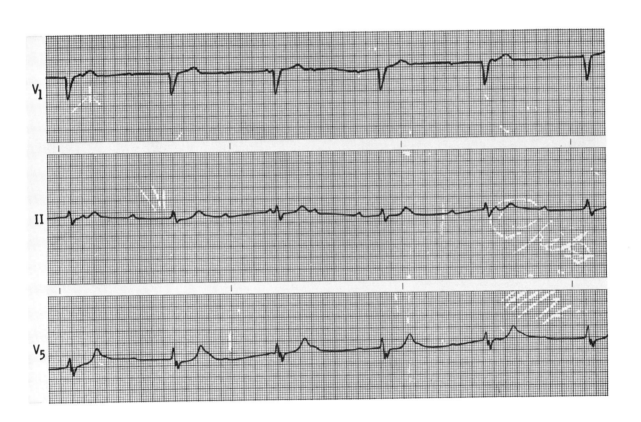

CASE 144: DIAGNOSIS

Arrows indicate the sinus P waves. The cardiac rhythm diagnosis is sinus rhythm (indicated by *arrows;* atrial rate 78 beats per minute) with ventricular escape (idioventricular) rhythm (ventricular rate 33 beats per minute) due to complete A-V block resulting in complete A-V dissociation. Note that the atrial and ventricular activities are entirely independent. In this case, the site of the block is in the infranodal region so that complete A-V block is due to complete trifascicular block (see Chapter 10).

In complete infranodal block, the escape impulses originate from the ventricles. Thus, the QRS complexes are usually broad and bizarre, and the ventricular rate is slower than 40 beats per minute in ventricular escape rhythm in most cases.

A permanent artificial pacemaker is definitely indicated for complete A-V block due to complete trifascicular block.

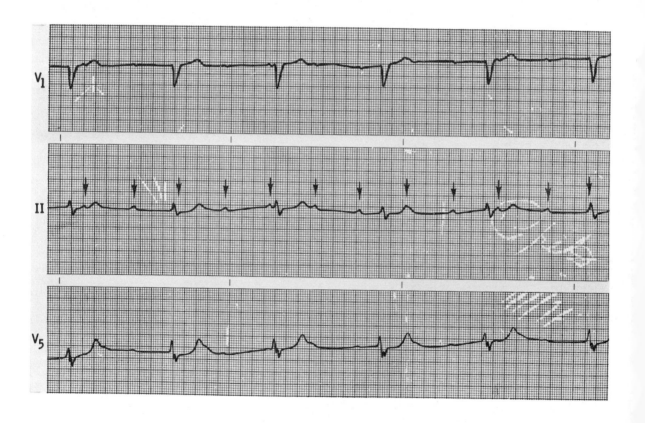

chapter 9

VENTRICULAR ARRHYTHMIAS

CASE 145

These cardiac rhythm strips were obtained from a 52-year-old man who has been experiencing palpitations.

1. *What is your cardiac diagnosis?*
2. *Is this cardiac arrhythmia a relatively benign or serious rhythm disorder?*

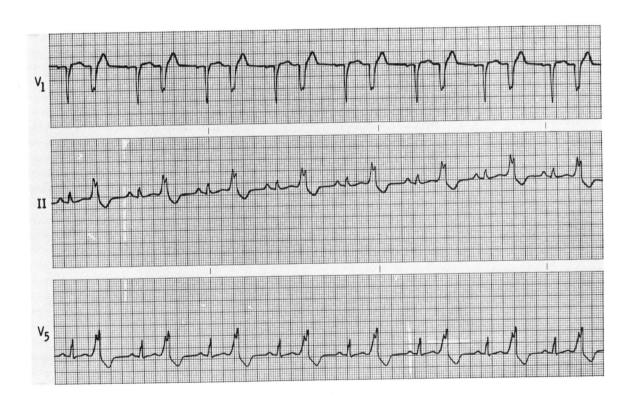

CASE 145: DIAGNOSIS

The basic cardiac rhythm is sinus (rate 100 beats per minute), but there are frequent ventricular premature contractions producing ventricular bigeminy. It should be noted that every other sinus P wave is superimposed on the QRS complexes of the ventricular premature contractions. This finding may lead to the erroneous diagnosis of sinus bradycardia as the underlying rhythm by recognizing every other sinus P wave.

As far as the configuration of the ventricular premature contractions is concerned, it shows left bundle branch block *pattern*. The left bundle branch block *pattern* of the ectopic beats means that the ventricular premature contractions originate from the right ventricle. On the other hand, left ventricular premature contractions reveal right bundle branch block pattern (see Case 146). When the QRS contour of the ventricular ectopic beats is primarily upright in both leads V_1 and V_5 and V_6, the ventricular premature contractions are considered to be arising from the cardiac apex or the ventricular septum (see Cases 147–149).

In general, right ventricular premature contractions as seen in this case are considered to be relatively benign, and they may be encountered in apparently healthy individuals. In contrast to this, ventricular premature contractions originating from the left ventricle or ventricular septum are nearly always found in patients with organic heart disease and/or digitalis intoxication.

Old diaphragmatic-lateral myocardial infarction is a remote possibility.

CASE 146

This electrocardiogram was obtained from a 56-year-old man with chronic congestive heart failure due to hypertensive heart disease. Digitalis intoxication was suspected.

1. *What is your cardiac rhythm diagnosis?*
2. *What is the drug of choice?*

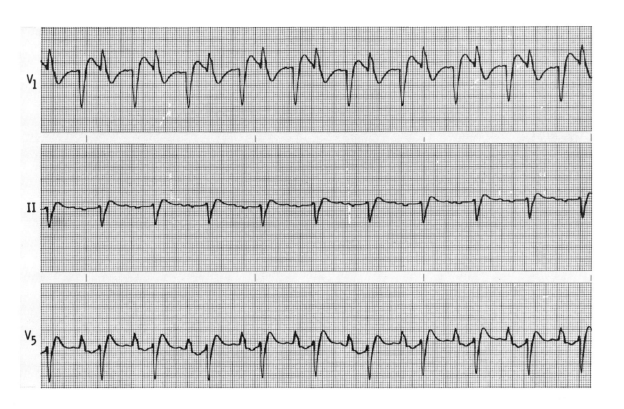

CASE 146: DIAGNOSIS

Arrows indicate sinus P waves. The cardiac rhythm is sinus tachycardia (atrial rate 125 beats per minute) with frequent ventricular premature contractions (marked *V*) producing ventricular bigeminy. Note that every other sinus P wave is superimposed on the QRS complexes of the ventricular premature contractions. By analyzing the contour of the ventricular ectopic beats, the left ventricular premature contractions can be diagnosed (see also Case 145).

In addition, there is left bundle branch block. Because of the pre-existing left bundle branch block, bidirectional ventricular tachycardia is closely simulated (see also Case 152).

As mentioned previously, digitalis-induced ventricular premature contractions commonly originate from the left ventricle as seen in this case.

The drug of choice for the digitalis-induced ventricular arrhythmias is diphenylhydantoin (Dilantin). When there is a significant hypokalemia, however, administration of potassium is also very effective. Dilantin may be given intravenously or orally, depending on the clinical circumstance. Needless to say, digitalis should be discontinued immediately before any drug therapy when digitalis intoxication is diagnosed.

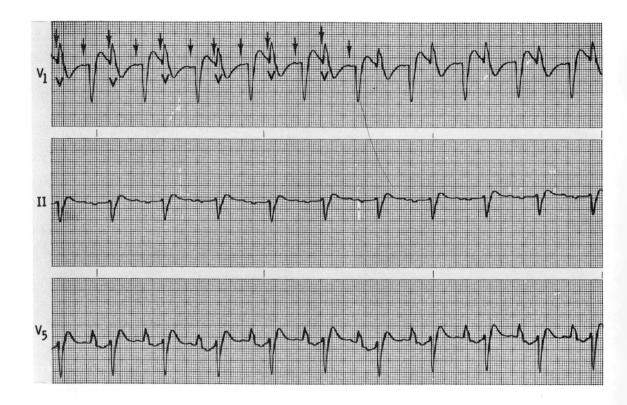

CASE 147

These cardiac rhythm strips were obtained from an 83-year-old woman with labile hypertension.

What is your cardiac rhythm diagnosis?

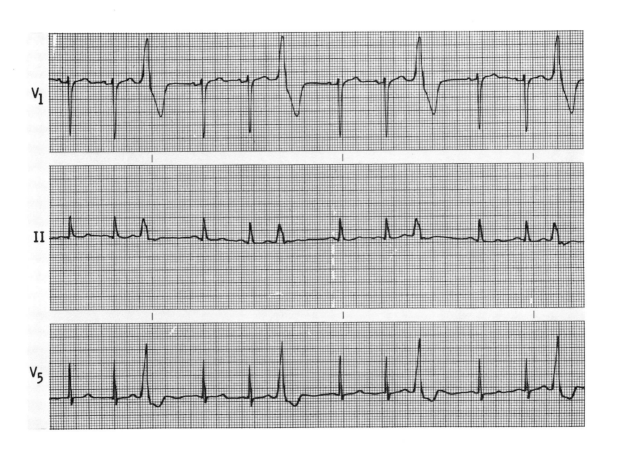

CASE 147: DIAGNOSIS

The underlying cardiac rhythm is sinus (rate 85 beats per minute), but there are frequent ventricular premature contractions which occur on every third beat—ventricular trigeminy.

Since the QRS configuration of the ventricular premature contractions demonstrate upright R waves in both leads V_1 and V_5 (right bundle branch block *pattern* in lead V_1, and left bundle branch block *pattern* in lead V_5), the ectopic focus is considered to be located in the ventricular septum. As indicated earlier (see also Case 145), ventricular premature beats arising from the left ventricle as well as the ventricular septum are observed commonly in elderly individuals and/or patients with organic heart disease.

CASE 148

A 77-year-old woman with severe angina pectoris was found to have irregular cardiac rhythm.

    1. What is your cardiac rhythm diagnosis?
    2. What is the other ECG abnormality?
    3. What is the drug of choice for this rhythm disorder?

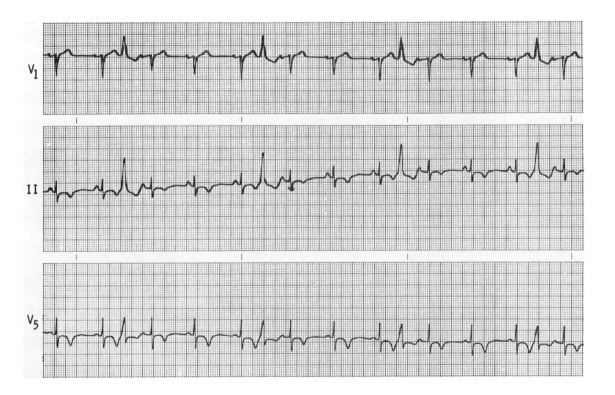

CASE 148: DIAGNOSIS

The basic cardiac rhythm is sinus (rate 73 beats per minute), but there are frequent ventricular premature contractions causing ventricular quadrigeminy. The ventricular premature contraction is not followed by a full compensatory pause. That is, the ventricular premature beat is sandwiched between two consecutive sinus beats. This finding is termed "interpolated" ventricular premature contraction.

By close observation, the R-R interval of two sinus beats containing a ventricular premature beat is found to be slightly longer than the remaining R-R intervals during sinus rhythm. This is due to the fact that the P-R interval of the sinus beat immediately following a ventricular premature contraction is prolonged as a result of a concealed ventriculoatrial conduction. In other words, a retrograde impulse from a ventricular premature contraction penetrates into the A-V junction leading to a longer refractory period of the A-V junction when the next sinus impulse is conducted to the ventricle. Since indirect evidence of the retrograde conduction from the ventricular ectopic beat into the A-V junction is observed in the following beat, the term "concealed" conduction is used. It should be noted that the sinus P-P cycles are *not* altered.

Another interesting finding is that the T wave configuration of the sinus beat immediately following a ventricular premature contraction is different from those of the remaining sinus beats. This T wave alteration is called "post-ectopic T wave change."

One of the important findings in the ventricular premature contractions is the duration of the coupling interval (the interval from the ectopic beat to the preceding beat of the basic rhythm). When the coupling interval is so short that the T wave of the preceding beat is interrupted by the ventricular premature beat, the threshold for the initiation of ventricular fibrillation becomes markedly reduced, leading to high incidence of ventricular fibrillation. This finding is termed the "R-on-T phenomenon" and requires immediate treatment.

This patient demonstrates frequent ventricular premature contractions with the "R-on-T phenomenon which should be treated. Lidocaine (Xylocaine) is usually effective for ventricular premature contractions found in coronary heart disease. Alternatively, propranolol (Inderal) may be tried for ventricular premature contractions associated with angina pectoris.

Her 12-lead ECG reveals T wave inversion involving practically all leads (only three leads are shown here) indicative of diffuse myocardial ischemia.

CASE 149

Digitalis intoxication was diagnosed in a 59-year-old man with chronic congestive heart failure due to hypertensive heart disease.

1. *What is your cardiac rhythm diagnosis?*
2. *What will be the best therapeutic approach for this patient?*

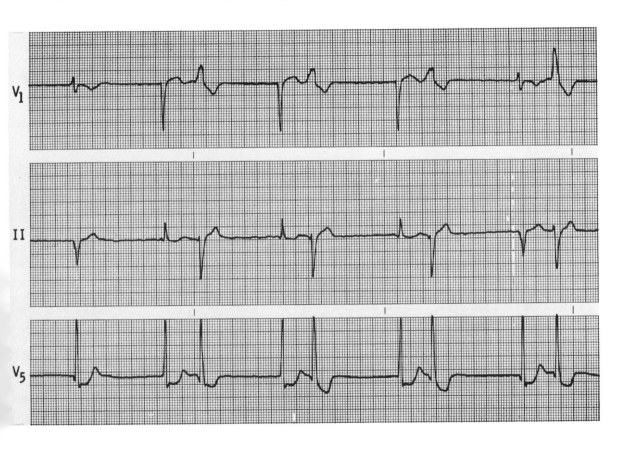

CASE 149: DIAGNOSIS

The underlying cardiac rhythm is atrial fibrillation, but the ventricular rate (rate 55–60 beats per minute) is slow, and there are three kinds of QRS complexes (marked *E, V,* and *X*). Thus, the cardiac rhythm diagnosis is atrial fibrillation with complete A-V block causing two types of escape beats: A-V junctional escape rhythm (marked *E*), as well as ventricular escape beats (marked *X*). In addition, there are frequent ventricular premature contractions (marked *V*) producing ventricular bigeminy. When dealing with this type of cardiac rhythm disorder, the diagnosis of a far-advanced digitalis intoxication is almost certain.

The use of a temporary artificial pacemaker with slight over-driving pacing rate should be considered when there are significant symptoms (*e.g.,* fainting, dizziness, hypotension, etc.) as a result of the cardiac arrhythmia itself. The over-driving pacing rate may be anywhere between 80–120 beats per minute, and the pacing should be sufficient to suppress the ventricular premature contractions. One or more antiarrhythmic agents, particularly diphenylhydantoin (Dilantin) and/or potassium may be added if the ventricular premature contractions are not suppressed by the over-driving pacing. Of course, digitalis should be discontinued immediately before any active treatment.

There is a clear evidence of left ventricular hypertrophy. In addition, old diaphragmatic myocardial infarction is a remote possibility.

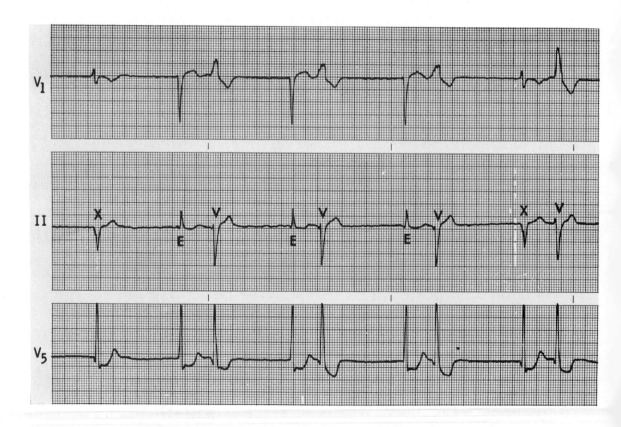

CASE 150

A 64-year-old woman was admitted to the Coronary Care Unit because of acute extensive anterior myocardial infarction (12-lead ECG taken on admission showed Q or Q-S waves in leads V_1 through V_6 with marked S-T segment elevation). She developed a rapid heart action soon after admission.

1. What is your cardiac rhythm diagnosis?
2. What is the best therapeutic approach?

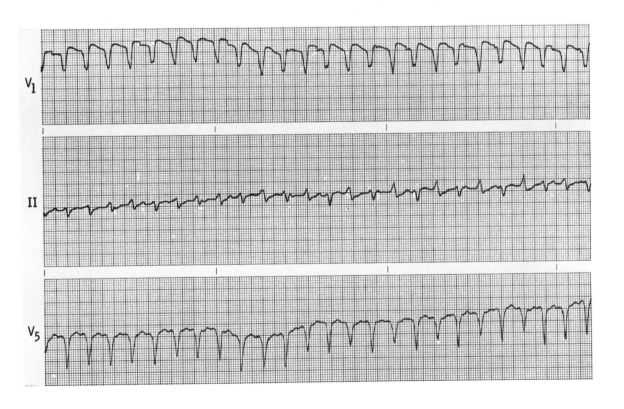

CASE 150: DIAGNOSIS

Arrows indicate sinus P waves. The cardiac rhythm reveals sinus tachycardia (indicated by *arrows;* atrial rate 118 beats per minute) with bidirectional ventricular tachycardia (ventricular rate 160 beats per minute) causing complete A-V dissociation. Note that the atrial and ventricular activities are independent throughout. The direct cause of A-V dissociation is, needless to say, ventricular tachycardia. The changing contour of the QRS complexes on every other beat during ventricular tachycardia is more clearly evident in lead II, and it is less pronounced in leads V_1 and V_5. Since the R-R intervals are regular, the bidirectional ventricular tachycardia is considered to be unifocal.

As far as the therapeutic approach is concerned, a direct current shock will be the treatment of choice if the clinical situation is extremely urgent (*e.g.,* the patient is hypotensive with or without fainting episodes or dizziness, etc.). Otherwise, intravenous injection of lidocaine (Xylocaine) will be the drug of choice. Following the termination of ventricular tachycardia, either by a direct current shock or intravenous injection of lidocaine, the patient should receive a continuous intravenous infusion (2–5 mg/min) of lidocaine for at least 24–72 hours.

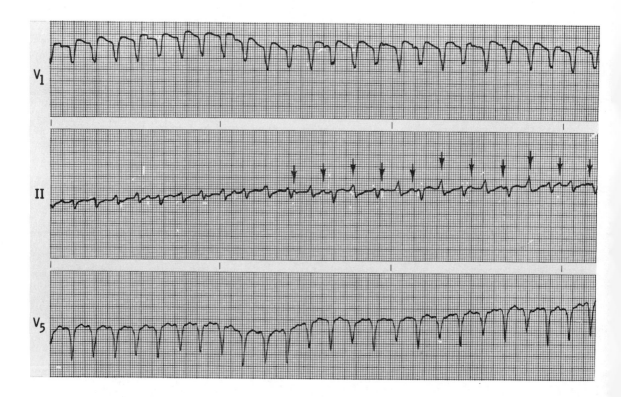

CASE 151

This electrocardiogram was obtained from a 34-year-old man with idiopathic cardiomyopathy. He was not taking any drug.

1. *What is your cardiac rhythm diagnosis?*
2. *What is the best therapeutic approach?*

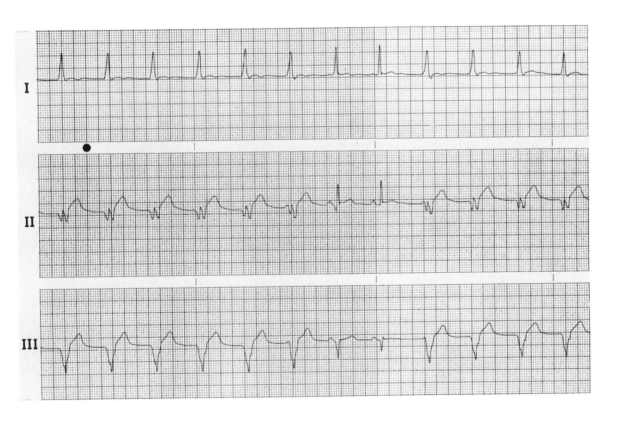

CASE 151: DIAGNOSIS

Arrows indicate sinus P waves. The underlying cardiac rhythm is sinus (indicated by *arrows*; atrial rate 82 beats per minute), but there are frequent bizarre beats. Thus, the cardiac rhythm diagnosis is sinus rhythm with intermittent parasystolic ventricular tachycardia (marked *V*; ventricular rate 80 beats per minute). Note a normally conducted sinus beat (marked *S*) as well as a ventricular fusion beat (marked *FB*). It should be recognized that the long interectopic interval containing sinus beats represents a multiple of the shortest interectopic intervals (ectopic ventricular cycles). The diagnostic criteria of parasystole have been described elsewhere (see Case 85).

As far as the clinical significance of parasystolic ventricular tachycardia is concerned, this arrhythmia is usually self-limited, and no treatment is necessary. Parasystolic ventricular tachycardia may be encountered in patients with various organic heart diseases. In addition, this arrhythmia may also occur in apparently healthy individuals. The most important clinical significance of parasystole is that this arrhythmia has never been reported as a digitalis-induced arrhythmia.

Abnormal Q waves were found in leads III and aVF (not shown here), but the finding is considered to be a pseudo-diaphragmatic myocardial infarction pattern.

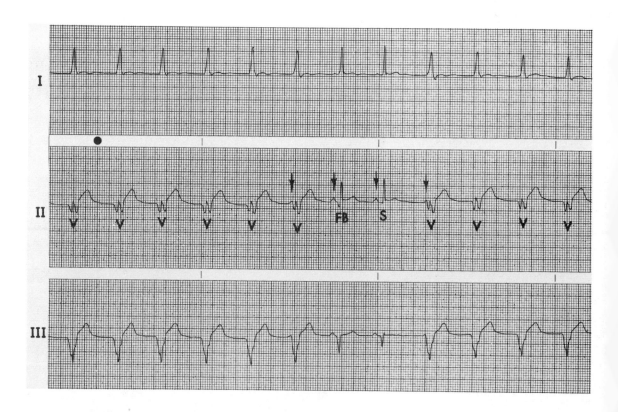

CASE 152

Digitalis intoxication was diagnosed in a 70-year-old man with cor-pulmonale and thyro-toxicosis. He expired soon after this ECG tracing was recorded.

What is your cardiac rhythm diagnosis?

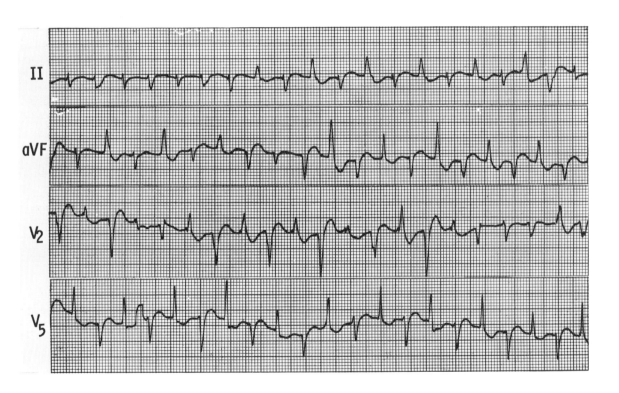

II

aVF

V₂

V₅

CASE 152: DIAGNOSIS

The cardiac rhythm discloses atrial fibrillation with bidirectional ventricular tachycardia (ventricular rate 167 beats per minute) producing complete A-V dissociation. In bidirectional ventricular tachycardia, the atrial mechanism is commonly ectopic rhythm including atrial fiibrillation, flutter, or tachycardia.

Clinically, the bidirectional ventricular tachycardia, especially in the presence of atrial tachyarrhythmia, is considered to be almost a pathognomonic feature of a far-advanced digitalis intoxication as seen in this case. Other causes of bidirectional ventricular tachycardia may include acute myocardial infarction (see Case 150) and cardiomyopathy. Bidirectional ventricular tachycardia may soon transform to ventricular fibrillation or flutter.

Bidirectional ventricular tachycardia is often irreversible in digitalis intoxication, and the serum digoxin level was more than 10 ng/ml (normal value 1.0–2.5 ng/ml) which is incompatible with life in most cases.

CASE 153

This electrocardiogram was obtained from a 56-year-old man with acute anterior myocardial infarction. He expired soon after this ECG tracing was recorded.

What is your cardiac rhythm diagnosis?

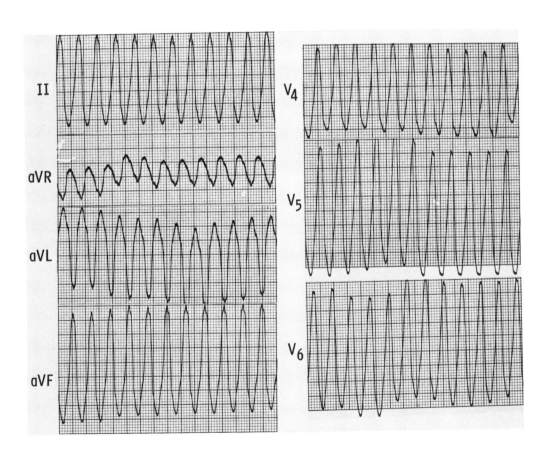

CASE 153: DIAGNOSIS

It is difficult to separate the S-T segment or T wave from the QRS complex in this ECG tracing. That is, the entire ECG complex appears to be a continuous loop. This kind of cardiac rhythm disorder is termed "ventricular flutter" (rate 215 beats per minute) which has the same clinical significance as ventricular fibrillation (see Case 154). In other words, the cardiac output becomes negligible or even near zero during ventricular flutter or fibrillation. Therefore, ventricular flutter should be terminated immediately by direct current shock. When the application of the direct current shock is delayed more than 4 minutes, irreversible brain damage is often unavoidable even if the cardiac function is restored later. After the termination of ventricular flutter, continuous intravenous infusion (2–5 mg/min) of lidocaine (Xyolcaine) is necessary for at least 24–72 hours in order to prevent the recurrence of the ventricular tachyarrhythmias.

CASE 154

These cardiac rhythm strips were obtained in the Coronary Care Unit from a 57-year-old man with massive acute anterior myocardial infarction. Leads II-a, b, and c are continuous.

What is your cardiac rhythm diagnosis?

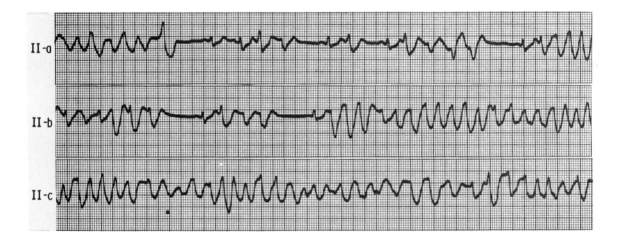

CASE 154: DIAGNOSIS

The basic cardiac rhythm is sinus tachycardia (rate 120 beats per minute) with frequent ventricular permature contractions which lead to ventricular fibrillation. Obviously, the R-on-T phenomenon with frequent ventricular premature beats initiates the ventricular fibrillation (see also Case 148). Note many isolated sinus beats between bouts of paroxysmal ventricular fibrillation in leads II-a and b.

Needless to say, immediate application of direct-current shock is mandatory for ventricular fibrillation. When ventricular fibrillation is not terminated within 4 minutes, the patient will suffer from permanent brain damage in most cases even if the sinus rhythm is restored later. It is recommended that every patient receive a continuous intravenous infusion (2–5 mg/min) of lidocaine (Xylocaine) for at least 24–72 hours following the termination of ventricular fibrillation.

chapter 10

INTRAVENTRICULAR CONDUCTION
DISTURBANCES

CASE 155

This electrocardiogram was obtained from a 76-year-old woman with coronary heart disease.

What is your ECG diagnosis?

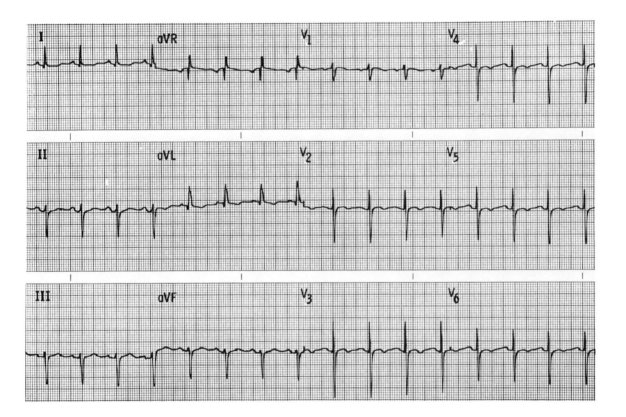

CASE 155: DIAGNOSIS

The cardiac rhythm discloses sinus rhythm with a rate of 97 beats per minute. It is easy to recognize marked left axis deviation of the QRS complexes (QRS axis −60°). This ECG finding represents left anterior hemiblock.

The diagnostic criteria of left anterior hemiblock are as follows:
1. Marked left axis deviation (QRS axis −45 to −90°).
2. Small q wave In lead I and small r wave in lead III.
3. Little or no prolongation of the QRS interval.
4. No evidence of other factors responsible for left axis deviation (true or pseudo).

The fundamental mechanism responsible for the production of marked left axis deviation in left anterior hemiblock is diagrammatically illustrated on this page. When both anterior and posterior divisions of left bundle branch system are intact (diagram *A*), the left ventricle is activated via both divisions (vectors 1 and 2) so that the resultant forces of vectors 1 and 2 will produce vector 3. When one of two divisions of the left bundle branch system is blocked, however, the impulses must travel through the intact division only. That is, anterior hemiblock (diagram *B*) vector 1 is no longer present, and as a result, the left ventricle is activated via intact posterior division (vector 2). In this case, the electrical axis shifts to the left and superiorly (marked left axis deviation). For the same reason, posterior hemiblock (diagram *C*) produces right axis deviation because the left ventricle is activated via intact anterior division (vector 1). **Key:** RB, right bundle branch block; AVN, A-V node; LAD, left anterior division; LPD, left posterior division.

As far as the clinical significance is concerned, left anterior hemiblock alone has no significance. Accordingly, no treatment is indicated. Chronic left anterior hemiblock is considered to be due to a sclerotic-degenerative process in the left anterior fascicle of the left bundle branch as seen in any other portion of the Purkinje system. However, left anterior hemiblock of acute onset is usually due to direct damage of the left anterior fascicle as a result of anteroseptal myocardial infarction.

The T waves are inverted in all precordial leads and the finding strongly suggests diffuse anterior myocardial ischemia.

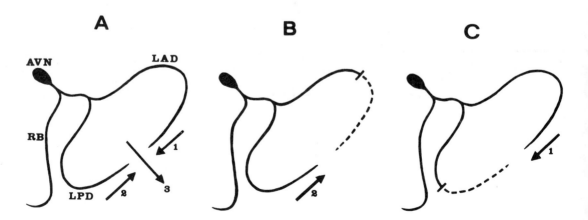

Diagram: Hemiblocks

CASE 156

A 46-year-old man was admitted to the Coronary Care Unit because of severe chest pain of 10–12 hours' duration.

1. *What is your ECG diagnosis?*
2. *What is the treatment of choice?*

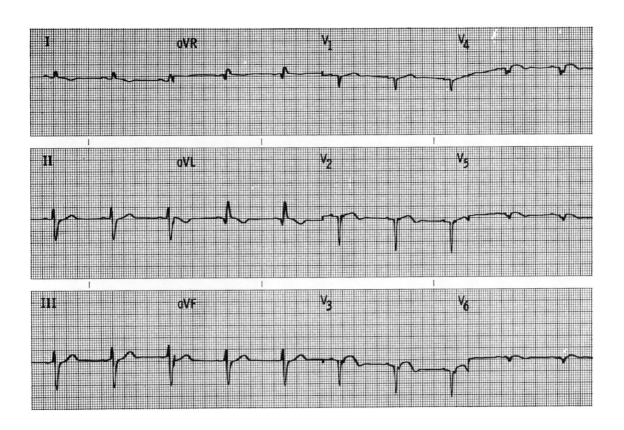

CASE 156: DIAGNOSIS

The cardiac rhythm is sinus with a rate of 62 beats per minute.

The diagnosis of acute extensive anterior myocardial infarction can be made without any difficulty (see Chapter 3). Another striking ECG abnormality is marked left axis deviation of the QRS complexes (QRS axis −65°) due to left anterior hemiblock (see Case 155). As indicated previously, left anterior hemiblock of acute onset is almost always produced by acute anterior myocardial infarction involving ventricular septum.

Left anterior hemiblock *per se* is clinically insignificant, and it requires no treatment. However, the patient should be observed closely for a possible development of a bifascicular or trifascicular block as a result of acute anterior myocardial infarction. For bifascicular or trifascicular block of acute onset as a result of acute anterior myocardial infarction (see Cases 164 and 166), an artificial pacemaker is considered to be indicated. It should be remembered that left anterior or posterior hemiblock may lead to Mobitz type-II A-V block or even complete A-V block as a result of a complete trifascicular block (see Case 167).

CASE 157

This ECG tracing was obtained from a 67-year-old woman with carcinoma of the breast. No evidence of organic heart disease was found.

What is your ECG diagnosis?

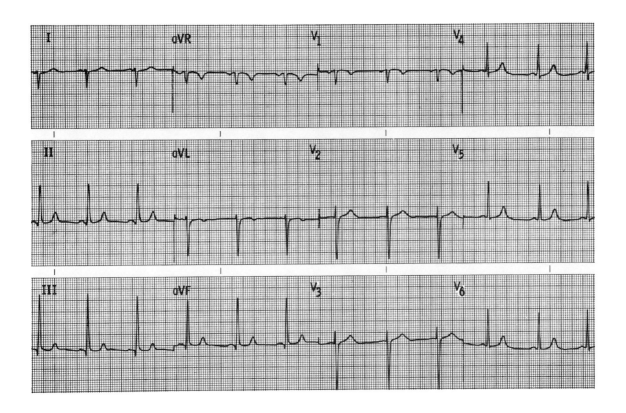

CASE 157: DIAGNOSIS

The cardiac rhythm is sinus with a rate of 68 beats per minute. This electrocardiogram appears to be normal except for the abnormal QRS axis. That is, the tracing reveals marked right axis deviation of the QRS complexes (QRS axis +105°) which represents left posterior hemiblock. The fundamental mechanism responsible for the production of right axis deviation in left posterior hemiblock has been described elsewhere (see Case 155).

The diagnostic criteria of left posterior hemiblock are summarized as follows:

1. Marked right axis deviation of the QRS complexes (axis +105 to +180°).
2. Small r wave in lead I and small q wave in lead III.
3. Little or no prolongation of the QRS interval.
4. No evidence of other factors responsible for right axis deviation of the QRS complexes (true or pseudo).

A pure form of left anterior hemiblock (see Cases 155 and 156) is much more common than left posterior hemiblock because of the following reasons. That is, the posterior division is shorter and thicker, and less influenced by the stresses of outflow pressure because of its inflow-tract structure. It also has a dual blood supply as compared with the anterior division.

Chronic left posterior hemiblock may be found in individuals with no apparent heart disease as seen in this case. However, left posterior hemiblock of acute onset is nearly always due to acute anteroseptal myocardial infarction, and the left posterior hemiblock often coexists with right bundle branch block (see Case 166). Otherwise, a bifascicular block consisting of left posterior hemiblock and right bundle branch block, with or without coexisting A-V block, is relatively common in patients with cardiomyopathy (see Case 165). A pure form of hemiblock may be found in calcific aortic stenosis or hypertensive heart disease. An isolated left posterior hemiblock requires no treatment.

CASE 158

A 21-year-old female student was seen at the Student Health Clinic for an annual physical checkup. She was found to be healthy, and no evidence of heart disease was appreciated.

What is your ECG diagnosis?

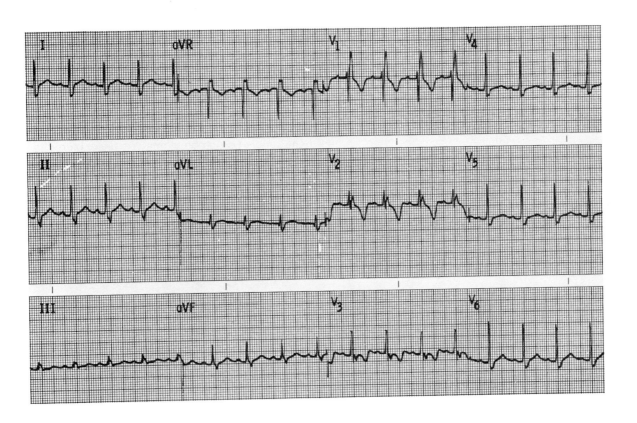

CASE 158: DIAGNOSIS

Cardiac rhythm is normal sinus rhythm with a rate of 100 beats per minute.

It is obvious that the QRS configuration is broad and bizarre. This QRS alteration is due to right bundle branch block. Namely, M-shape pattern (RR′ complex) of the QRS complexes is observed in leads V_1 and V_2 with slurred and deep S waves in leads I, II, aVL, aVF, and V_4 through V_6. In addition, there is T wave inversion in leads V_1 through V_3, as a manifestation of the secondary T wave change. These ECG abnormalities are the characteristic features of right bundle branch block as a result of a delayed activation in the right ventricle due to a block at the right bundle branch system. It should be noted that the initial ventricular septal activation in right bundle branch block is normal.

The diagnostic criteria of right bundle branch block are summarized as follows:

1. M pattern or rSR′ pattern of the QRS complex in leads V_1 through V_3.
2. Deep and slurred S waves in leads I, aVL, and V_4 through V_6.
3. Broad QRS interval 0.12 second or more.
4. Secondary S-T, T wave changes in leads V_1 through V_3.

The term "incomplete" right bundle branch block is used when the QRS interval is less than 0.12 second (0.09–0.11 second).

As far as the clinical significance is concerned, right bundle branch block may be encountered in apparently healthy individuals as seen in this case. On the other hand, atrial septal defect should be always considered in any individuals, particularly in children and young adults, with unexplainable right bundle branch block (see Cases 27 and 141). In addition, right bundle branch block with acute onset may be due to pulmonary embolism (see Case 197). Right bundle branch block may also develop suddenly in patients with acute anteroseptal myocardial infarction (see Case 162). Right bundle branch block often coexists with left anterior or posterior hemiblock causing a bifascicular block (see Cases 163–166).

CASE 159

These cardiac rhythm strips were obtained from a 53-year-old man with coronary heart disease. He gave a history of "heart attack" 6 months previously. He has been taking pro-pranolol (Inderal) (20 mg) 4 times daily.

What is your ECG diagnosis?

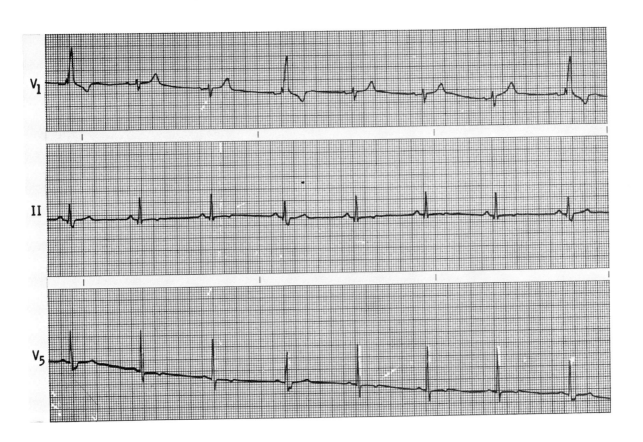

CASE 159: DIAGNOSIS

The cardiac rhythm discloses sinus bradycardia with a rate of 48 beats per minute.

There are three bizarre and broad QRS complexes because of intermittent right bundle branch block. Ventricular premature contractions are closely simulated.

His 12-lead ECG (not shown here) demonstrated evidence of diaphragmatic and posterior myocardial infarction. The R wave in lead V_1 is relatively tall with tall and symmetric upright T wave as a result of posterior myocardial infarction (see Chapter 3).

Inderal was prescribed for his angina following myocardial infarction, and sinus bradycardia in this case is due to Inderal effect.

CASE 160

This electrocardiogram was obtained from a 62-year-old man with hypertensive heart disease.

What is your ECG diagnosis?

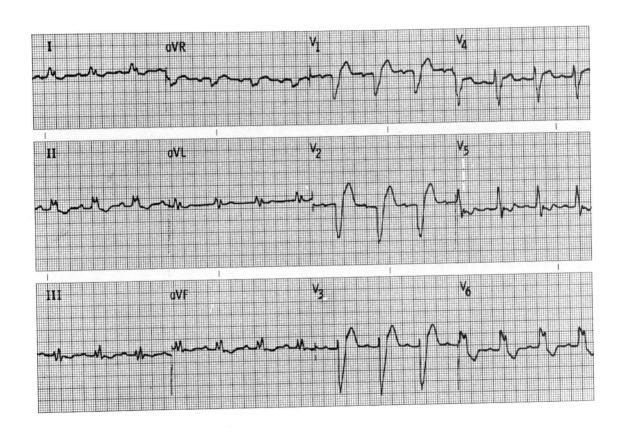

CASE 160: DIAGNOSIS

The cardiac rhythm is sinus (rate 85 beats per minute) with first degree A-V block (P-R interval 0.22 second).

It is apparent that the QRS interval is broad and the configuration is bizarre (M shape in many leads, particularly in leads I and V_6). In addition, the T waves are inverted or biphasic in leads I, II, III, aVF, and V_5 and V_6 with S-T segment depression as a manifestation of the secondary S-T, T wave change. These ECG findings are the characteristic features of left bundle branch block.

The diagnostic criteria of left bundle branch block are summarized as follows:

1. M (rsR′) pattern or broad R waves in leads I, aVL, and V_4 through V_6.
2. Broad Q-S or rS waves in leads V_1 through V_3 (sometimes up to leads V_4 and V_5).
3. Absence of the physiologic septal q waves in leads I, aVL, and V_4 through V_6.
4. The broad QRS interval 0.12 second or more.
5. Secondary S-T, T wave change in leads I, aVL, and V_4 through V_6.

The term "incomplete" left bundle branch block is used when the QRS interval is less than 0.12 second. It is important to remember that leads V_1 through V_3 (sometimes up to leads V_4 and V_5) may show Q-S waves (absence of r waves) in a pure left bundle branch block. This ECG finding obviously mimics anteroseptal myocardial infarction. However, the Q-S waves in leads V_1 through V_3 in left bundle branch block are simply due to the alteration of the initial ventricular septal force. In other words, the initial septal force may be directed posteriorly and to the left in approximately one-third of a pure left bundle branch block.

As far as the clinical significance is concerned, left bundle branch block is most commonly found in hypertensive heart disease. The second most common underlying disease is probably aortic stenosis. Other causes of left bundle branch block may include coronary artery disease, cardiomyopathy, and other various heart diseases. Anatomically, the majority of patients with left bundle branch block demonstrate evidence of left ventricular hypertrophy. It is extremely unusual to observe left bundle branch block in healthy individuals with no demonstrable heart disease.

CASE 161

These ECG rhythm strips were obtained from a 30-year-old man with aortic stenosis.

What is your ECG diagnosis?

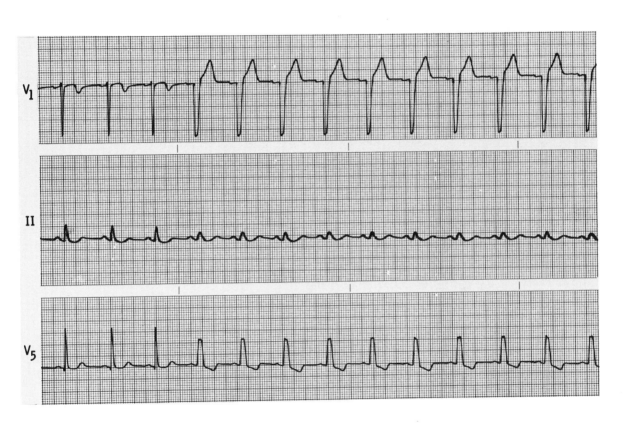

CASE 161: DIAGNOSIS

The cardiac rhythm is sinus rhythm with a rate of 80 beats per minute. There are two types of QRS complexes because of intermittent left bundle branch block. The cardiac rhythm during left bundle branch block closely mimics ectopic rhythm such as nonparoxysmal ventricular tachycardia (accelerated ventricular rhythm) or parasystolic ventricular tachycardia (see Case 151).

The term "rate-dependent" bundle branch block is used when right or left bundle branch block occurs during faster ventricular rate. Otherwise, intermittent bundle branch block is said to be "rate-independent" as seen in this case. In general, rate-dependent bundle branch block eventually becomes rate-independent bundle branch block which finally leads to a fixed and chronic bundle branch block.

As indicated earlier, left bundle branch block is common in patients with aortic stenosis.

CASE 162

A 68-year-old woman was admitted to the Coronary Care Unit because of severe chest pain of several hours' duration. In reviewing her previous ECG tracings before this admission, no ECG abnormality was found.

> 1. What is your ECG diagnosis?
> 2. Is artificial pacing indicated?

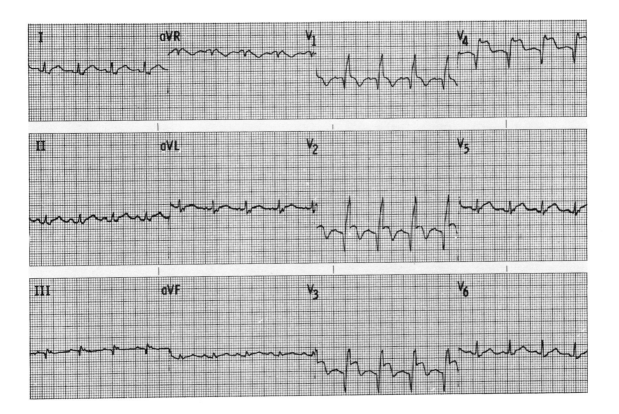

CASE 162: DIAGNOSIS

The cardiac rhythm is sinus tachycardia with a rate of 106 beats per minute.

The diagnosis of right bundle branch block can be made on the basis of the diagnostic criteria described in Case 158. However, it becomes obvious that there is another coexisting ECG abnormality. That is abnormal Q waves with S-T segment elevation and T wave inversion in leads V_1 through V_4 indicative of acute anteroseptal myocardial infarction (see Chapter 3). In addition, the QRS amplitude is markedly diminished in the limb leads—low voltage, which is very common in acute myocardial infarction (see also Case 32). Old diaphragmatic myocardial infarction is a remote possibility.

This patient developed right bundle branch block suddenly as a result of acute anteroseptal myocardial infarction. Although there is a significant controversy regarding the use of an artificial pacemaker in acute myocardial infarction, prophylactic artificial pacing is considered to be *not* indicated for right bundle branch block due to myocardial infarction.

When the patient develops a bifascicular or trifascicular block as a result of acute myocardial infarction, however, the artificial pacemaker is considered to be indicated (see Cases 164 and 166).

CASE 163

A 53-year-old man was referred to a cardiologist because of an abnormal electrocardiogram. He denied any symptom such as fainting episodes, dizziness, or slow pulse rate. He had been apparently healthy all his life.

1. *What is your ECG diagnosis?*
2. *What is the appropriate diagnostic approach?*
3. *What is the appropriate therapeutic approach?*

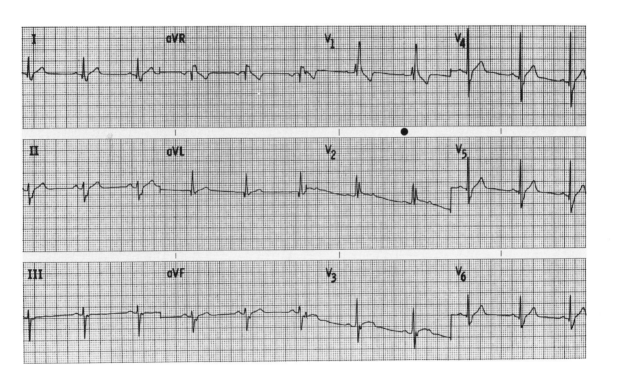

CASE 163: DIAGNOSIS

The cardiac rhythm is sinus with a rate of 62 beats per minute.

It is readily recognized that the QRS configuration is broad and bizarre due to right bundle branch block (see Case 158). Another ECG abnormality is marked left axis deviation of the QRS complexes (QRS axis −70°) as a result of left anterior hemiblock (see Case 155). Thus, a combination of right bundle branch block and left anterior hemiblock represents a bifascicular block which is a form of incomplete bilateral bundle branch block.

Although this patient seems to be asymptomatic from the bifascicular block, it is preferable to obtain a 24-hour Holter monitor (ambulatory) electrocardiogram. This is necessary because any patient with incomplete bilateral bundle branch block may develop intermittent complete bilateral bundle branch block causing complete A-V block or Mobitz type-II A-V block. When any patient with a bifascicular or trifascicular block demonstrates intermittent Mobitz type-II A-V block or complete A-V block even momentarily and even without significant symptom, a permanent artificial pacemaker implantation is mandatory.

In addition, the His bundle electrocardiogram has great value to predict the potential development of a complete A-V block. It has been shown that there is a high incidence of complete A-V block in the near future when the H-V interval (the interval from the His bundle potential to the ventricular deflection) is more than 70 msec in a patient with a bifascicular block. Therefore, many cardiologists recommend the prophylactic artificial pacing for patients with a bifascicular block associated with prolonged H-V interval. However, this view is not uniformly accepted.

The prophylactic pacing is *not* considered for asymptomatic patients with a chronic bifascicular block alone. The therapeutic approach for a bifascicular or trifascicular block with acute onset as a result of acute anterior myocardial infarction is different from that of chronic bifascicular or trifascicular block (see Cases 164 and 166).

CASE 164

A 64-year-old man was admitted to the Coronary Care Unit because of severe chest pain with acute onset. There was no history of a fainting episode, although he was in shock on admission.

1. What is your ECG diagnosis?
2. Is artificial pacing indicated?

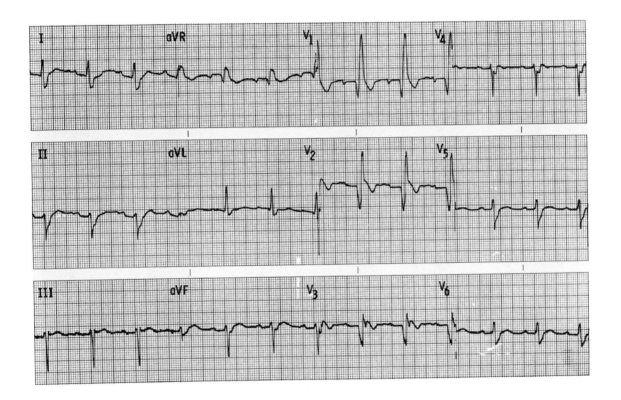

CASE 164: DIAGNOSIS

The cardiac rhythm is sinus rhythm (rate 75 beats per minute) with first degree A-V block (P-R interval 0.26 second).

The diagnosis of a bifascicular block can be made without any difficulty on the basis of a combination of right bundle branch block and left anterior hemiblock (see Cases 155 and 158). Incomplete trifascicular block is strongly suggested because there is a combination of first degree A-V block and the bifascicular block.

Another striking ECG abnormality is acute anteroseptal myocardial infarction (abnormal Q waves in leads V_1 through V_3 with S-T segment elevation and T wave inversion).

This patient developed a bifascicular block associated with first degree A-V block (suggestive of incomplete trifascicular block) acutely as a result of acute anteroseptal myocardial infarction. The prophylactic artificial pacing is recommended for any patient with a bifascicular or incomplete trifascicular block as a result of acute anteroseptal myocardial infarction in the hope that the potential development of Adams-Stokes syndrome or even sudden death due to complete A-V block can be prevented.

Left atrial hypertrophy is suggested (see Case 11).

CASE 165

This ECG tracing was obtained from a 75-year-old man with cardiomyopathy. He denied fainting episodes, lightheadedness, or a history of "heart attack."

1. What is your ECG diagnosis?
2. Is artificial pacing indicated?

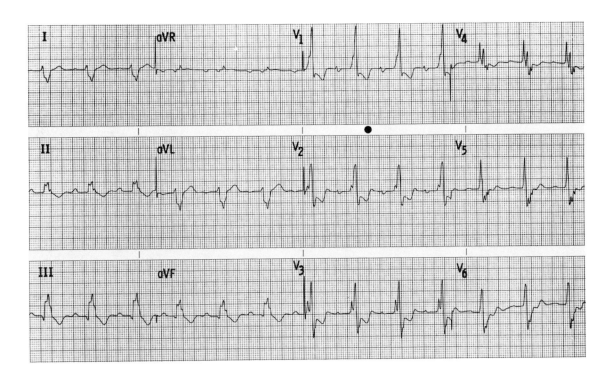

CASE 165: DIAGNOSIS

The cardiac rhythm is sinus (rate 75 beats per minute) with first degree A-V block (P-R interval 0.26 second).

It is easy to recognize the evidence of a bifascicular block which consists of right bundle branch block and left posterior hemiblock (QRS axis +120°). Thus, the diagnosis of incomplete trifascicular block is strongly suggested on the basis of a combination of first degree A-V block and the bifascicular block. In addition, there are Q waves in leads III and aVF suggestive of diaphragmatic myocardial infarction, but the finding is considered to be a pseudo-infarction pattern which is relatively common in patients with cardiomyopathy. Another ECG abnormality is left atrial hypertrophy (see Case 11).

As far as the therapeutic approach is concerned, prophylactic artificial pacing is considered to be *not* indicated for asymptomatic chronic bifascicular or incomplete trifascicular block. The prophylactic pacing may be considered, however, when the patient demonstrates the evidence of second degree (usually Mobitz type-II) or complete A-V block on other occasions, or the H-V interval is significantly prolonged (more than 70 msec) on the His bundle electrocardiogram.

CASE 166

This electrocardiogram was obtained from a 76-year-old man with recent myocardial infarction. There was no history of fainting episodes.

1. What is your ECG diagnosis?
2. Is artificial pacing indicated?

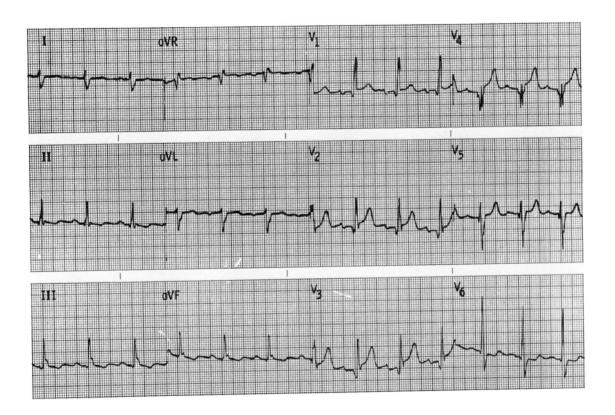

CASE 166: DIAGNOSIS

The cardiac rhythm is sinus (rate 74 beats per minute) with slight first degree A-V block (P-R interval 0.22 second).

A bifascicular block is diagnosed on the basis of right bundle branch block associated with left posterior hemiblock (QRS axis +115°). Another ECG abnormality is acute anteroseptal myocardial infarction. In addition, there is an evidence of left atrial hypertrophy. Left ventricular hypertrophy is also suggested.

This patient developed the bifascicular block acutely as a result of anteroseptal myocardial infarction.

The prophylactic artificial pacing is recommended for all patients with a bifascicular or incomplete trifascicular block due to acute anteroseptal myocardial infarction.

CASE 167

These cardiac rhythm strips were obtained from a 55-year-old woman with Adams-Stokes syndrome. Leads II-a, b, c, and d are continuous.

1. *What is your ECG diagnosis?*
2. *What is the treatment of choice?*

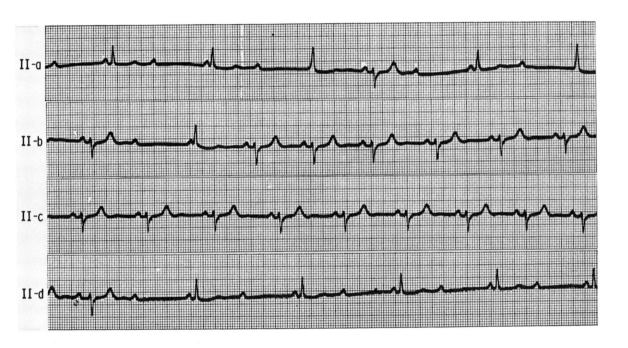

CASE 167: DIAGNOSIS

Arrows indicate sinus P waves. The cardiac rhythm is sinus rhythm (indicated by *arrows;* atrial rate 70 beats per minute) with intermittent complete A-V block causing areas (leads II-a and d) of ventricular escape (idioventricular) rhythm (ventricular rate 37 beats per minute).

As far as the configuration of the QRS complexes during normal sinus rhythm (leads II-b and c) is concerned, it shows marked left axis deviation (QRS axis −50°, calculated from a 12-lead ECG) indicative of left anterior hemiblock. Thus, intermittent complete A-V block in this case is considered to be a manifestation of incomplete trifascicular block. In some areas such as lead II-d, 2:1 A-V block is closely simulated. Intermittent complete A-V block is called high degree (advanced) A-V block.

Permanent artificial pacemaker implantation is the treatment of choice for symptomatic bifascicular or trifascicular block, particularly when advanced A-V block (intermittent complete A-V block) is documented on other occasions.

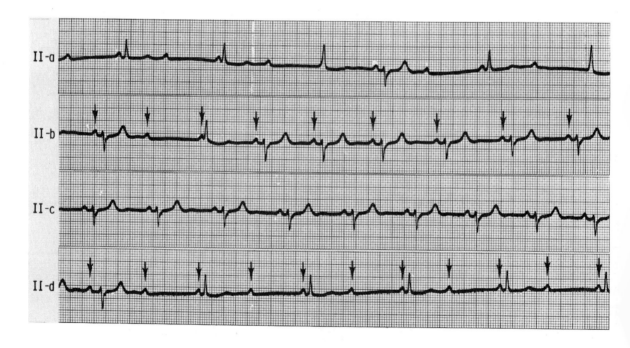

chapter 11

WOLFF-PARKINSON-WHITE (WPW) SYNDROME

CASE 168

This electrocardiogram was obtained from a 31-year-old man with frequent episodes of palpitations.

What is your ECG diagnosis?

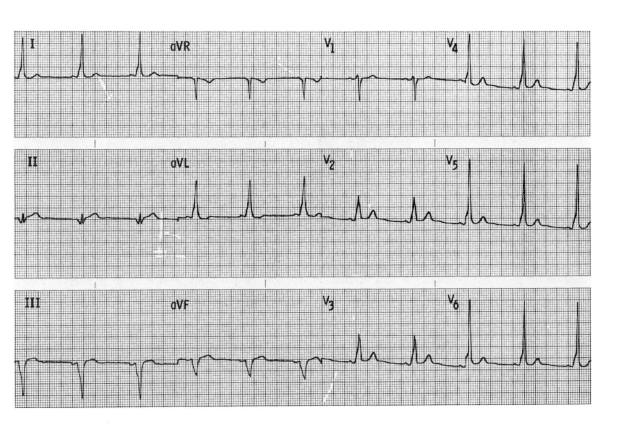

CASE 168: DIAGNOSIS

The cardiac rhythm is sinus rhythm (rate 60 beats per minute) with left axis deviation of the P wave (P axis −30°). As indicated earlier (see Case 8), left axis deviation of the sinus P wave (P axis ranging from 0 to −60°) may occur in apparently healthy individuals. When the P axis is beyond −60° (−60 to −90°), the P wave is considered to be a retrograde P wave as seen in A-V junctional beats or rhythm (see Chapter 7).

The striking ECG abnormality in this tracing is a short P-R interval (P-R interval 0.08 second) with borad QRS complex (QRS interval 0.14 second) due to initial slurring of the QRS complex. These ECG findings are the characteristic features of the Wolff-Parkinson-White (WPW) syndrome. The initial slurring of the QRS complex is often called "delta wave" which is considered to be due to a premature activation of a portion of the ventricles as a result of anomalous A-V conduction via an accessory pathway.

The diagnostic criteria of the WPW syndrome are summarized as follows:

1. Initial slurring (delta wave) of the QRS complex.
2. Short P-R interval.
3. Prolonged QRS interval.
4. Secondary T wave change (not always present).

Among the above diagnostic criteria, the most important finding is the initial slurring (delta wave) of the QRS complex which is responsible for a short P-R interval and a broad QRS complex.

It is important to recognize that leads II, III, and aVF demonstrate Q or Q-S waves diagnostic for diaphragmatic myocardial infarction (see Chapter 3). However, this ECG finding is a pseudo-dia-phragmatic myocardial infarction pattern as a result of delta waves which are directed superiorly. In addition, a pseudo-left ventricular hypertrophy pattern is also present.

The fundamental mechanism responsible for the production of a unique ECG finding in the WPW syndrome is diagrammatically illustrated. Uninterrupted line indicates anomalous conduction in WPW syndrome; dotted line indicates normal conduction. P-R and P-R′ intervals are A-V con-duction times in WPW syndrome and normal conduction, respectively. P-R interval is shorter than P-R′ interval due to delta wave. Note that P-Z and P-S intervals are constant during anomalous and normal conduction. T wave in WPW syndrome is inverted because of secondary T wave change.

Needless to say, the most important clinical significance of the WPW syndrome is the extremely high incidence (50–75%) of various supraventricular tachyarrhythmias (see Cases 174–176). He was found to have frequent episodes of reciprocating tachycardia (see Case 174) which required propranolol (Inderal).

Although a precise classification of the WPW syndrome is not possible in every case, the syn-drome has been classified into two groups, type-A and B, depending on the direction of delta wave (see Case 169).

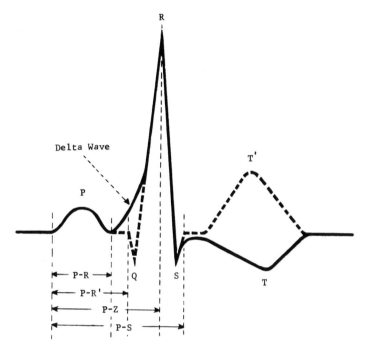

WOLFF-PARKINSON-WHITE SYNDROME

CASE 169

A 48-year-old apparently healthy woman was referred to a cardiologist for the evaluation of frequent episodes of palpitations.

What is your ECG diagnosis?

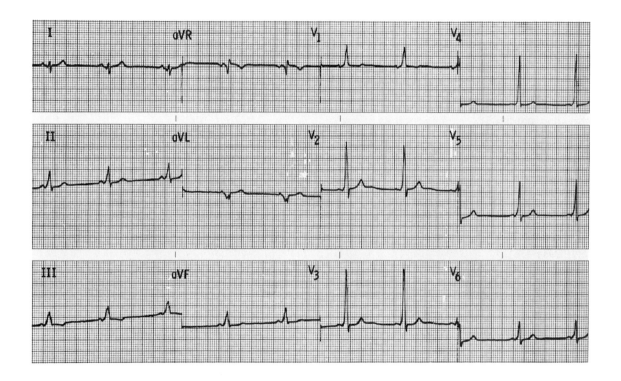

CASE 169: DIAGNOSIS

The cardiac rhythm is sinus bradycardia with a rate of 57 beats per minute.

The diagnosis of the WPW syndrome, type A is readily made on the basis of a short P-R interval (P-R interval 0.08 second) and a broad QRS complex (QRS interval 0.12 second) due to a delta wave (see Case 168). The delta wave is directed anteriorly so that the QRS complexes are primarily upright in all precordial leads. This ECG finding closely mimics right bundle branch block, right ventricular hypertrophy, and posterior and high lateral (Q or Q-S wave—negative delta waves in leads I and aVL) myocardial infarction.

As far as the classification of the WPW syndrome is concerned, the syndrome has been customarily divided into two groups, type-A and B. The classification has been made simply according to the QRS configuration in the precordial leads.

In type-A, the premature component and the remainder of the QRS complex are primarily upright in both left and right precordial leads (leads V_1 through V_6) as seen in this case (see also Cases 171 and 176). In general, lead V_1 shows R, RS, Rs, RSr' and Rsr' patterns, while leads V_5 and V_6 show Rs or R complex. In a practical sense, type A WPW syndrome can be diagnosed without any difficulty when the QRS complexes are primarily upright in all precordial leads as seen in this case, providing that the ECG tracing is taken correctly.

In type-B, the left precordial leads (leads V_4 through V_6) show tall R waves with delta waves, and leads V_1 and V_2 reveal delta waves with negative QRS complexes. Thus, leads V_1 and V_2 often show rS or Q-S pattern in type-B WPW syndrome (see Cases 168 and 170).

Nevertheless, the above classification is clearly arbitrary because some of the cases of WPW syndrome cannot be classified simply to either type-A or B. In addition, the classification from the vectorial approach is somewhat different from the electrocardiographic classification. Vectorcardiographically, the delta wave is directed anteriorly in type-A, whereas it is directed posteriorly in type-B. In either type-A or B WPW syndrome, the delta wave may be directed either superiorly or inferiorly. If we follow the vectorial classification, a pure type-B WPW syndrome is extremely rare (see Case 170).

It should be recognized that in type-A WPW syndrome, the premature activation occurs in the left ventricle via anomalous A-V conduction. On the other hand, in type-B WPW syndrome, the premature activation occurs in the right ventricle.

In addition to frequent occurrence of pseudo-diaphragmatic myocardial infarction pattern in both type-A and B WPW syndrome, many other ECG abnormalities are often closely simulated. Type-A WPW syndrome closely mimics right bundle branch block, right ventricular hypertrophy and a true posterior myocardial infarction (see Cases 169, 171, and 176). On the other hand, type-B WPW syndrome produces a pseudo-left bundle branch block pattern, a pseudo-left ventricular hypertrophy pattern and a pseudo-anteroseptal myocardial infarction pattern (see Cases 168 and 170).

CASE 170

This electrocardiogram was obtained from an 11-year-old girl with paroxysmal rapid heart action.

What is your ECG diagnosis?

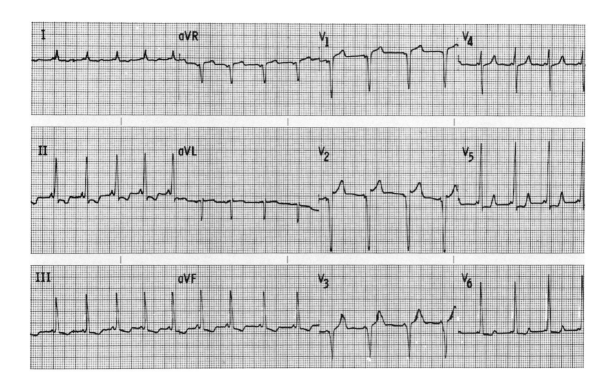

CASE 170: DIAGNOSIS

The cardiac rhythm is sinus arrhythmia with areas of sinus tachycardia with rate ranging from 86–115 beats per minute.

The diagnosis of the WPW syndrome, type-B is obvious (see Cases 168 and 169). In fact, the ECG finding in this tracing is a typical example of WPW syndrome, type-B either by electrocardiographic or vectorcardiographic classification criteria (see Case 169).

The Q-S pattern in leads V_1 through V_3 closely resembles anteroseptal myocardial infarction, and tall R waves with the secondary S-T, T wave change in leads V_4 through V_6 closely mimic left ventricular hypertrophy.

CASE 171

This ECG tracing was obtained from a 35-year-old woman with repetitive episodes of palpitation. Propranolol (Inderal) was effective in preventing the rapid heart action.

What is your ECG diagnosis?

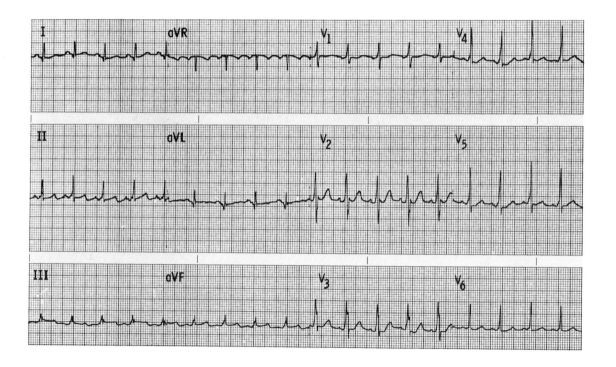

CASE 171: DIAGNOSIS

The cardiac rhythm is sinus tachycardia with a rate of 112 beats per minute.

At a glance, the diagnosis of the WPW syndrome is *not* obvious because the QRS complex is not significantly prolonged. However, a close observation enables one to recognize the delta waves resulting in short P-R intervals and broad QRS complexes. Thus, this ECG tracing demonstrates the WPW syndrome, type-A (see Cases 168 and 169).

It is important to understand that the delta wave is not obvious in every case of the WPW syndrome. The location of the accessory pathway is primarily responsible for the duration of the delta wave. In other words, the delta wave is pronounced when the accessory pathway connecting the atria and ventricles is far away from the normal A-V conduction system. In contrast to this, the delta wave is not obvious when the accessory pathway is very near to the normal A-V conduction system. The term "Lown-Ganong-Levine (LGL) syndrome" has been used when the delta wave is not clearly shown so that the ECG tracing appears to show a short P-R interval and apparently normal QRS complex associated with rapid heart action. By reviewing the literature concerning so-called LGL syndrome, it is simply a variant of the WPW syndrome in many cases.

Regarding the P-R interval in the WPW syndrome, a short P-R interval is *not* an absolute criterion because a delayed A-V conduction may coexist with the syndrome.

CASE 172

These cardiac rhythm strips were obtained from a 12-year-old girl. Leads II-a, b, c, and d are continuous.

What is your ECG diagnosis?

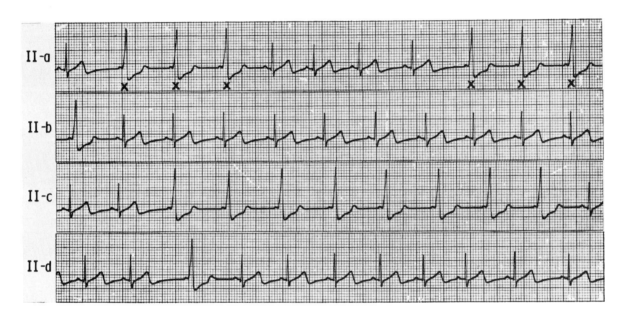

CASE 172: DIAGNOSIS

The cardiac rhythm reveals sinus arrhythmia with rate ranging from 75–96 beats per minute.

It is obvious that there are two kinds of QRS complexes. Namely, this ECG tracing shows intermittent WPW syndrome (marked X) which seems to occur during slower heart rate. Intermittent WPW syndrome closely resembles nonparoxysmal ventricular tachycardia (accelerated ventricular rhythm) or parasystolic ventricular tachycardia (see Case 151). Otherwise, intermittent WPW syndrome (marked X) superficially simulates intermittent left bundle branch block (see Case 161).

CASE 173

The Holter monitor (ambulatory) electrocardiogram was obtained from a 24-year-old man because he complained of frequent episodes of rapid heart action. Many 12-lead electrocardiograms were taken previously on this patient, but no ECG abnormality was documented. The rhythm strips *A* to *D* are not continuous, and they represent lead II.

What is your ECG diagnosis?

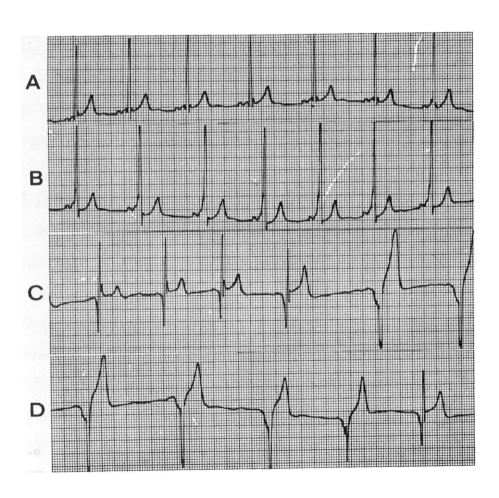

CASE 173: DIAGNOSIS

It is apparent that there are four kinds of QRS complexes. The basic cardiac rhythm is sinus arrhythmia and areas of sinus bradycardia with rate ranging from 43–62 beats per minute.

Not only the WPW syndrome is intermittent, but also there are the WPW complexes with three kinds of anomalous A-V conduction. Strip *A* shows normal A-V conduction except for the last beat. The remaining rhythm strips *B, C,* and *D* demonstrate a triple anomalous A-V conduction. Multiple anomalous conduction in the WPW syndrome has been reported previously by different authors, and anatomic documentation of the multiple accessory conduction pathways has also been reported.

CASE 174

A bout of rapid heart action was recorded from a 48-year-old woman with proven WPW syndrome, type A.

    1. What is your cardiac rhythm diagnosis?
    2. What is the drug choice?

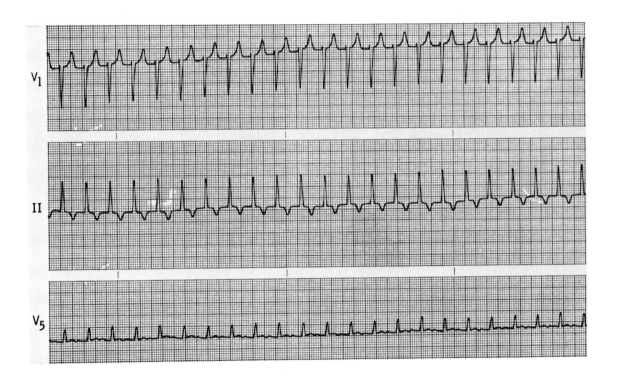

CASE 174: DIAGNOSIS

The cardiac rhythm reveals a regular tachycardia (rate 143 beats per minute) with normal QRS complexes without discernible P waves. No delta wave is appreciated. This type of tachycardia has been called "supraventricular tachycardia" without specifying the exact location of the ectopic impulse formation. On the other hand, the term "paroxysmal atrial tachycardia" or "A-V junctional tachycardia" have been also used to designate the same finding.

From the electrophysiologic investigation, however, the regular tachycardia in the WPW syndrome as seen in this case was proven to be a reciprocating (re-entrant or circus-movement) tachycardia due to a specific re-entry phenomenon via normal and anomalous pathways.

The fundamental mechanism responsible for the production of the reciprocating tachycardia in the WPW syndrome is described as follows:

Diagram (Part I) illustrating the mechanism of a reciprocating tachycardia with normal QRS complex in WPW syndrome. In diagram A, atrial premature impulse (marked A) is conducted to the A-V node (marked N), but the atrial premature impulse is blocked in the anomalous pathway. The atrial premature impulse is then conducted to both ventricles via bundle branch system (diagram A). In diagram B, the atrial impulse is conducted to the atria in retrograde fashion to produce an inverted P wave. In diagram C, the impulse is conducted in a clockwise fashion producing reciprocating (re-entry) cycle, and the same cycle may repeat indefinitely. Note that the QRS complex during the tachycardia is normal. **Key:** S, sinus node; d, delta wave; P, inverted P wave.

Diagram (Part II) illustrating a reciprocating tachycardia with anomalous conduction in WPW syndrome. The re-entry cycle is in a counter-clockwise fashion which is exactly the reverse of that shown in Diagram (Part I).

It has been shown that a reciprocating tachycardia is the most common tachyarrhythmia associated with the WPW syndrome, and the majority of cases show normal QRS complexes. Less commonly, atrial fibrillation may be observed (see Case 176), and atrial flutter is extremely rare (see Case 175) in the WPW syndrome. In both atrial fibrillation and flutter, the QRS complexes are almost always bizarre because of anomalous A-V conduction and/or aberrant ventricular conduction due to extremely rapid ventricular rate (see Cases 175 and 176).

The drug of choice is propranolol (Inderal) for a reciprocating tachycardia with normal QRS complexes. Digitalis is equally effective under this circumstance.

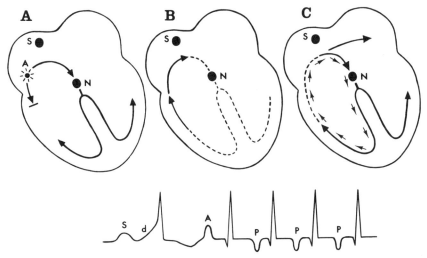

Reciprocating tachycardia in WPW syndrome
Diagram (Part I): Normal QRS complex

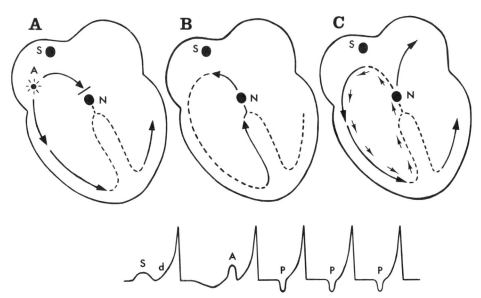

Reciprocating tachycardia in WPW syndrome
Diagram (Part II): Abnormal QRS complex (anomalous AV conduction)

CASE 175

A 78-year-old man was brought to the emergency room because of extremely rapid heart action (tracing A). He was not taking any drug. The ECG (tracing B) shown on the next page was taken after the termination of the rapid heart action.

1. *What is your cardiac rhythm diagnosis (tracing A)?*
2. *What is the treatment of choice (tracing A)?*
3. *What is the underlying disorder responsible for the production of this rapid heart action (tracing A)?*
4. *What other ECG abnormality is present?*

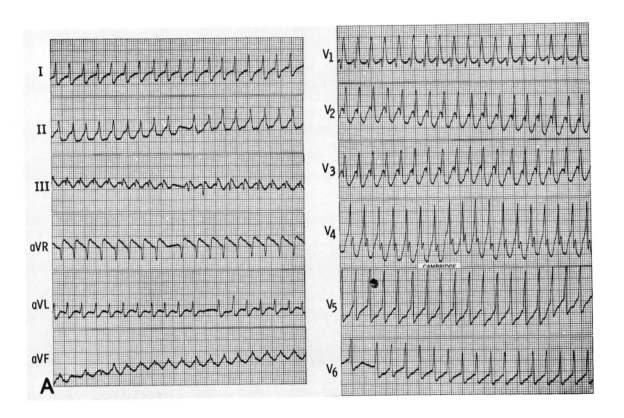

CASE 175: DIAGNOSIS

The cardiac rhythm exhibits a regular tachycardia with occasional ventricular pauses, and the rate is extremely fast (rate 250 beats per minute) with bizarre QRS complexes. By close observation, one can appreciate that the ventricular pause is shorter than two basic ventricular cycles. Therefore, this ECG tracing shows atrial flutter (atrial rate 250 beats per minute) with 1:1 A-V conduction (see also Case 96) and intermittent slowly progressing Wenckebach A-V conduction.

The bizarre QRS complexes are due to two factors; namely, anomalous A-V conduction because of the WPW syndrome and coexisting right bundle branch block. The diagnosis of the WPW syndrome and right bundle branch block is obvious on tracing B during sinus rhythm.

As far as the therapeutic approach is concerned, immediate application of direct current shock is the treatment of choice when the clinical situation is urgent. Direct current shock is extremely effective for atrial flutter and a small energy (10–50 wsec) discharge is sufficient. When the clinical situation is not extremely urgent, however, intravenous injection (50–100 mg) of lidocaine (Xylocaine) is considered to be the drug of choice for tachyarrhythmias, particularly atrial flutter or fibrillation, with anomalous A-V conduction in the WPW syndrome. As preventive measures, quinidine or procainamide (Pronestyl) by mouth are considered to be the agents of choice under this circumstance.

Propranolol (Inderal) or digitalis is ineffective for tachyarrhythmias with anomalous A-V conduction because these agents have no effect on the anomalous conduction in the WPW syndrome. In addition, digitalis is considered to be relatively contraindicated because the drug may accelerate the anomalous A-V conduction leading to a deterioration of the clinical circumstance. Furthermore, ventricular fibrillation may be produced under this circumstance, and sudden death may be unavoidable in some cases.

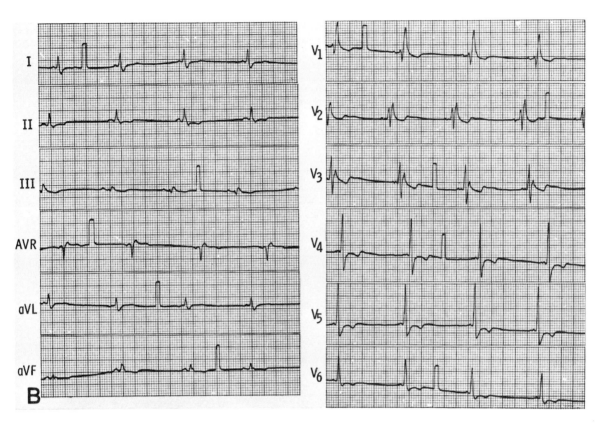

CASE 176

A 24-year-old healthy man developed rapid heart action (tracing A). He had suffered from similar episodes previously. Tracing B was taken following the termination of the rapid heart action.

1. What is your cardiac rhythm diagnosis (tracing A)?
2. What is the underlying disorder responsible for the production of this rapid heart action?
3. What is the treatment of choice?

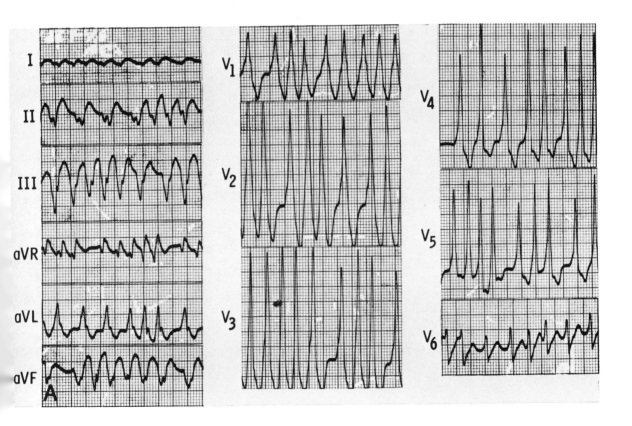

CASE 176: DIAGNOSIS

In tracing A, the cardiac rhythm appears to be ventricular tachycardia or even ventricular fibrillation. However, the correct diagnosis is atrial fibrillation with anomalous A-V conduction due to the WPW syndrome, type-A. The ventricular rate is extremely rapid (rate 180–300 beats per minute), and the QRS configuration is broad and bizarre. The diagnosis of the WPW syndrome, type-A is obvious during sinus rhythm (tracing B).

The treatment of choice is the immediate application of direct current shock (100–200 wsec). When the clinical situation is not extremely urgent, intravenous injection (50–100 mg) of lidocaine (Xylocaine) is the agent of choice. For prevention of this tachyarrhythmia, oral quinidine or procainamide (Pronestyl) are the drugs of choice.

Propranolol (Inderal) is totally ineffective in this case. In addition, digitalis is not only ineffective, but also the drug often enhances the anomalous A-V conduction leading to deterioration of the clinical outcome. In fact, this patient developed a true ventricular fibrillation soon after the administration of digitalis, but fortunately, defibriilator was applied immediately and sinus rhythm was restored (tracing B).

Note a psuedo-diaphragmatic and posterior myocardial infarction pattern during sinus rhythm because of the WPW syndrome, type-A (tracing B).

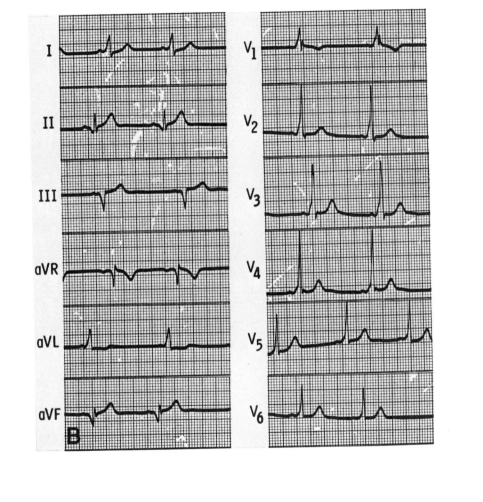

chapter 12

ARRHYTHMIAS RELATED TO ARTIFICIAL PACEMAKERS

CASE 177

These rhythm strips were obtained from a 69-year-old woman with previous history of a "heart attack," following implantation of a permanent artificial pacemaker.

1. *What is your cardiac rhythm diagnosis?*
2. *What is the other ECG abnormality?*

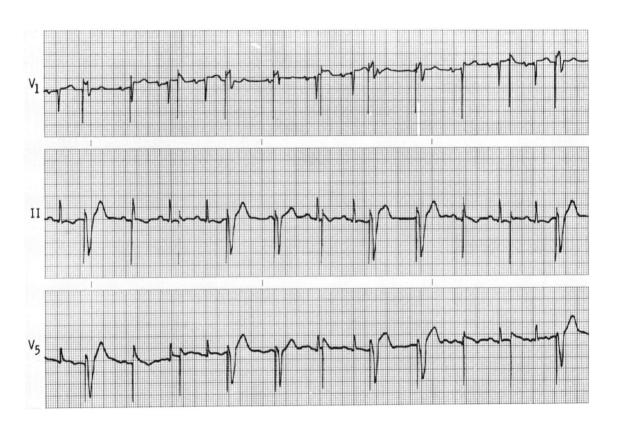

CASE 177: DIAGNOSIS

The underlying cardiac rhythm is sinus rhythm with a rate of 95 beats per minute. In addition to the basic sinus rhythm, there are regularly occurring artificial pacemaker spikes with intermittent ventricular capture. Because of the nature of the fixed-rate ventricular pacemaker, the basic sinus rhythm and the artificial pacemaker-induced ventricular rhythm compete with each other. Note occasional ventricular fusion beats (third and seventh beats). Because of a competition between two rhythms, the R-on-T phenomenon (see Case 148) is frequently observed. It has been shown that a sudden death is approximately 5 times more common in patients with a fixed-rate ventricular pacemaker than in patients with a demand pacemaker. This is considered to occur because of the development of ventricular fibrillation as a result of the R-on-T phenomenon.

It is well documented that normal A-V conduction occurs from time to time in 25% of patients with well-established complete A-V block. Therefore, a demand pacemaker is superior than a fixed-rate pacemaker, and recently, the former has gradually replaced the latter in most medical institutions.

There is evidence of diaphragmatic-lateral myocardial infarction which had occurred 6 months previously.

CASE 178

A 41-year-old woman developed a slowing of the pulse rate during digitalization. Digitalis toxicity was diagnosed, and a temporary artificial pacemaker was inserted.

What is your cardiac rhythm diagnosis?

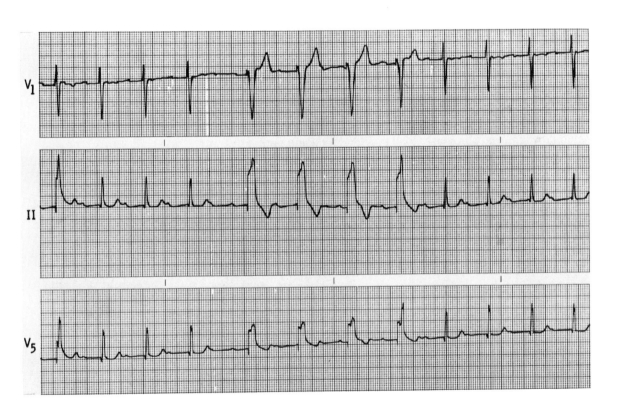

CASE 178: DIAGNOSIS

Arrows indicate ectopic P waves. The underlying cardiac rhythm is atrial tachycardia (atrial rate 165 beats per minute) with varying degree A-V block and areas of advanced (high-degree) A-V block. Advanced A-V block is responsible for the slowing of the ventricular rate for which a temporary (demand) artificial pacemaker was inserted. There are five artificial pacemaker-induced ventricular beats (marked X) during high-degree A-V block. The fact that atrial tachycardia associated with varying degree A-V block is almost a pathognomonic feature of digitalis toxicity has been emphasized previously (see Case 92).

By superficial examination, the underlying cardiac rhythm in this tracing appears to be sinus rhythm with first degree A-V block when the ectopic P waves are not recognized.

It is interesting to note that the pacing interval from the QRS complex of the basic rhythm to the next pacing beat is longer than the consecutively occurring pacing intervals. This finding is called "pacemaker hysteresis." A detailed description of pacemaker hysteresis is found elsewhere (see Case 191).

In most cases with digitalis-induced advanced or complete A-V block, a temporary (demand) artificial pacemaker is sufficient in addition to discontinuation of digitalis.

It is important to remember that the demand pacemaker is designed to function only when the natural rhythm becomes slower than the pre-set pacing rate.

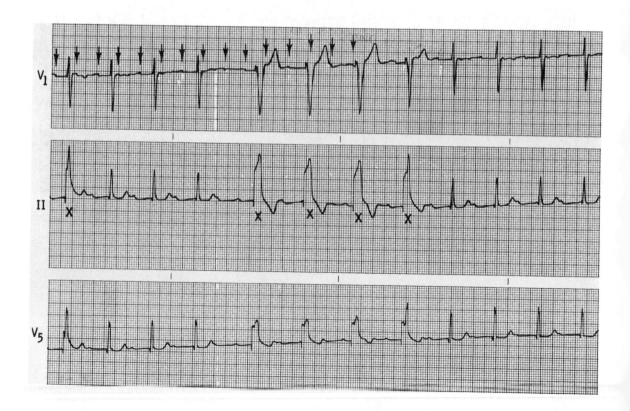

CASE 179

This electrocardiogram was obtained from a 69-year-old man with extensive anterior myocardial infarction.

What is your cardiac rhythm diagnosis?

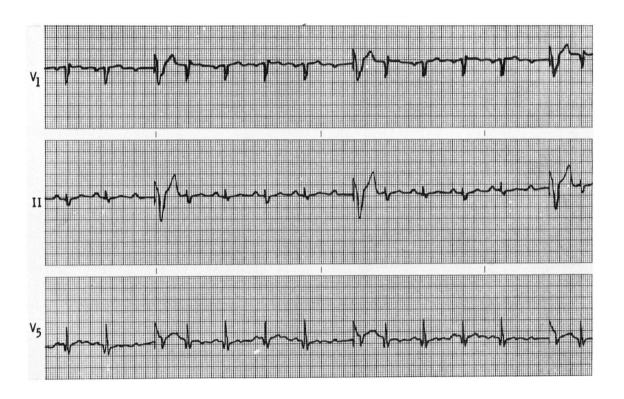

CASE 179: DIAGNOSIS

The underlying cardiac rhythm is sinus rhythm with a rate of 84 beats per minute. It should be noted that there is intermittent Mobitz type-II A-V block which leads to occasional occurrence of the demand pacemaker beats (3rd, 8th, and 13th QRS complexes).

As described previously, Mobitz type-II A-V block is considered to be a precursor of complete A-V block, and the block is in the infranodal region (see Case 136).

Mobitz type-II A-V block is always produced by irreversible damage in the Purkinje system, and the A-V block is often due to anterior myocardial infarction involving ventricular septum. Because of the irreversible damage in the conduction system, permanent artificial pacemaker implantation is indicated. Mobitz type-II A-V block is almost always associated with bundle branch block or bifascicular block, and the P-R intervals remain constant in all conducted beats.

In this tracing, there is evidence of right bundle branch block associated with extensive anterior myocardial infarction (Q or Q-S waves in leads V_2 through V_6 with embryonic r wave in lead V_1—only 3 leads are shown here).

CASE 180

A temporary artificial pacemaker was inserted in an 87-year-old woman with coronary heart disease because of intermittent slow heart rate associated with lightheadedness and hypotension.

What is your cardiac rhythm diagnosis?

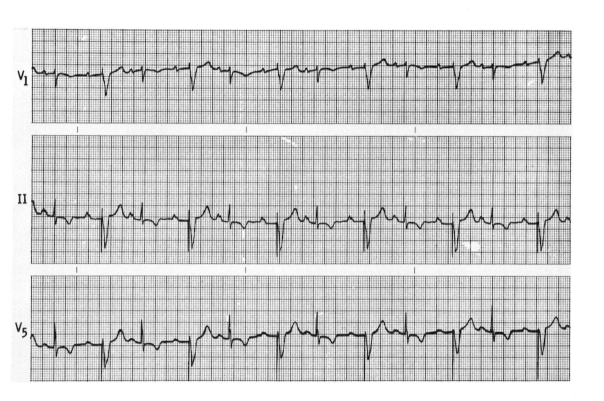

CASE 180: DIAGNOSIS

The underlying cardiac rhythm is sinus rhythm (atrial rate 78 beats per minute) with 2:1 A-V block. It is readily recognized that the demand pacemaker-induced ventricular beats occur when the sinus P waves are not conducted to the ventricles. As a result, the sinus beats and the pacemaker beats occur alternately, causing a form of ventricular bigeminy. This finding can be called a "demand pacemaker escape-bigeminy" which is analogous to A-V junctional escape-bigeminy (see Case 77) or ventricular escape-bigeminy (see Case 137).

As indicated earlier, 2:1 A-V block may be a variant of either Mobitz type-I or II A-V block, but a variant of Wenckebach (Mobitz type-I) A-V block is the most likely diagnosis when the QRS complexes of the sinus beats show a normal configuration (see Case 134).

This patient developed advanced A-V block intermittently, and a demand pacemaker was inserted.

The T waves are inverted practically in all leads (only 3 leads are shown here) indicative of diffuse myocardial ischemia.

CASE 181

A 43-year-old man developed ventricular tachycardia associated with recent myocardial infarction. A temporary artificial pacemaker was inserted because the ventricular tachycardia became refractory to various antiarrhythmic agents.

  1. *What is your cardiac rhythm diagnosis?*
  2. *What is the ECG abnormality?*

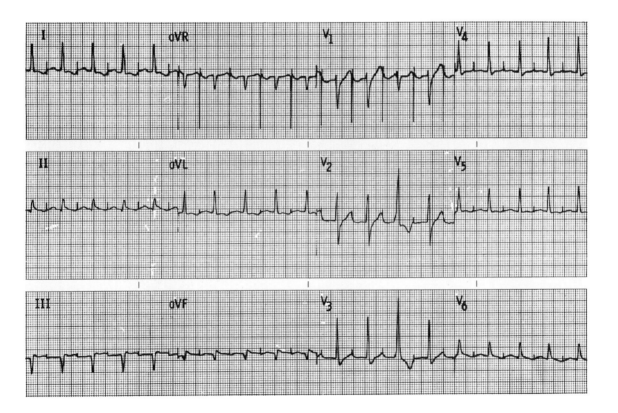

CASE 181: DIAGNOSIS

The cardiac rhythm is an over-driving atrial pacemaker rhythm with a rate of 112 beats per minute. Note that each pacemaker spike is followed by the P wave, which is similar to the ordinary sinus P wave, and a constant P-R interval. This finding indicates that the right atrium is stimulated by an artificial pacemaker. The over-driving pacing (rate 112 beats per minute) was successful in suppressing ventricular tachycardia. There is a ventricular premature contraction (13th beat).

It is easy to recognize the evidence of recent diaphragmatic-lateral myocardial infarction (abnormal Q waves in leads II, III, aVF, and V_6). In addition, posterior myocardial ischemia is suggested on the basis of relatively tall T waves in leads V_1 and V_2.

CASE 182

This electrocardiogram was obtained from a 36-year-old man with angina pectoris who required a temporary artificial pacemaker for marked sinus bradycardia.

What is your cardiac rhythm diagnosis?

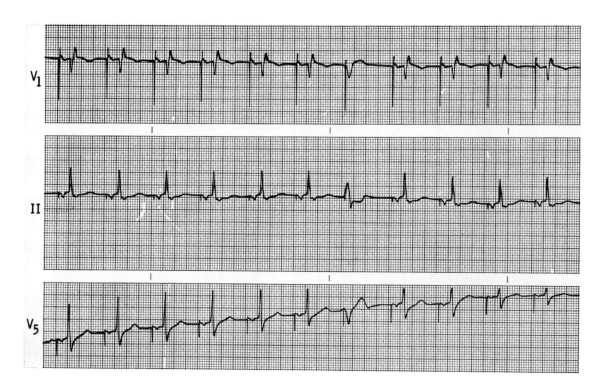

CASE 182: DIAGNOSIS

The cardiac rhythm reveals coronary sinus pacemaker rhythm with a rate of 75 beats per minute. Note that each pacemaker spike is followed by a retrograde P wave and the P-R interval is constant. The P-R interval in the coronary sinus pacemaker rhythm depends on the status of the A-V conduction system in a given patient. The QRS complex in the coronary sinus pacemaker rhythm, of course, is identical to the sinus beat in a given patient. Note a ventricular premature contraction (seventh beat).

The advantage of the coronary sinus pacemaker is similar to that of the atrial synchronized pacemaker (see Case 183). That is, the atrial contribution is utilized, and the normal atrioventricular as well as intraventricular conduction sequence is observed.

There is evidence of right bundle branch block.

CASE 183

These rhythm strips were obtained from a 43-year-old woman. Leads II-a and b are not continuous.

What is your cardiac rhythm diagnosis?

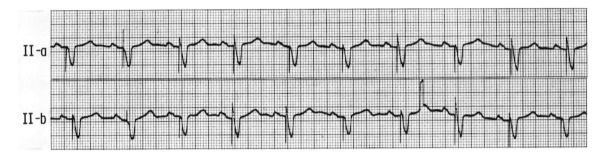

CASE 183: DIAGNOSIS

The caridac rhythm is atrial synchronized pacemaker rhythm with a rate of 74 beats per minute. The atrial synchronized pacemaker has many other names including synchronous pacemaker, Nathan pacemaker, and atrial-triggered pacemaker.

The atrial synchronized pacemaker is a more physiologic type of pacemaker, and the pulse generator is triggered by the natural P wave of atrial depolarization. Following the atrial depolarization, the ventricular stimulation occurs after an optimal delay corresponding to the P-R interval. In other words, an atrial synchronized pacemaker functions as an electronic bundle of His.

The major advantage of this type of pacemaker is its ability to provide maximum augmentation of the cardiac output at changing atrial rates to meet varying physiologic requirements. Another benefit is the utilization of the atrial contribution to ventricular filling to further augment the cardiac output. Thus, the atrial synchronized pacemaker becomes extremely valuable in younger or more active individuals. When atrial tachycardia or flutter occurs, the pacemaker induces A-V block of varying degree so that an optimum ventricular rate is maintained.

An atrial synchronized pacemaker is contraindicated in atrial fibrillation, marked sinus bradycardia, unstable sinus activity such as S-A block or sinus arrest and atrial standstill.

CASE 184

These cardiac rhythm strips were obtained from a 60-year-old woman with coronary heart disease.

What is your cardiac rhythm diagnosis?

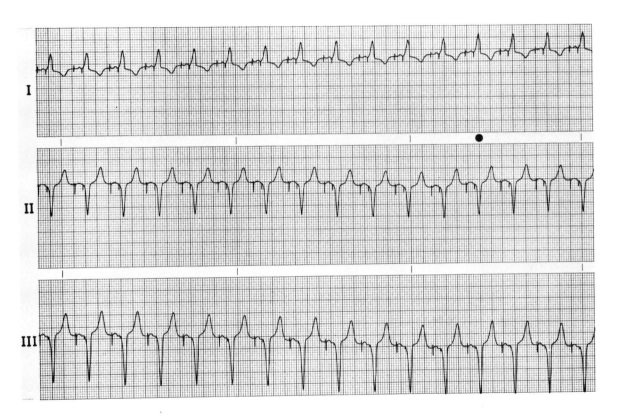

CASE 184: DIAGNOSIS

The cardiac rhythm discloses a bifocal demand pacemaker rhythm with a rate of 97 beats per minute. It should be noted that there are two sets of artificial pacemaker spikes, one of which initiates the P wave, whereas the other set initiates the QRS complex with constant P-R interval.

The bifocal (sequential atrioventricular) demand pacemaker consists of two demand units—a conventional QRS-inhibited ventricular pacemaker and a QRS-inhibited atrial pacemaker. In this model, the escape interval of the atrial pacemaker is designed to be shorter than that of the ventricular pacemaker; therefore the difference between these two escape intervals is a determining factor for the A-V sequential delay. The bifocal demand pacemaker may be able to stimulate both atria and ventricles in sequence, or stimulate the atria alone, or remain totally dormant so that the pacemaker functions automatically according to the individual patient's need.

In general, the bifocal demand pacemaker is considered to be indicated in the following situations:

1. Sick sinus syndrome.
2. Significant atrial bradyarrhythmias associated with intermittent high-degree or complete A-V block (symptomatic).
3. High-degree or complete A-V block (symptomatic) in that atrial contribution to the ventricular output is essential.

The bifocal demand pacemaker does not compete with spontaneous ventricular contractions.

CASE 185

These rhythm strips were obtained from a 64-year-old woman following permanent artificial pacemaker implantation. An artificial pacemaker was implanted in this patient because of Adams-Stokes syndrome due to complete A-V block.

What is your cardiac rhythm diagnosis?

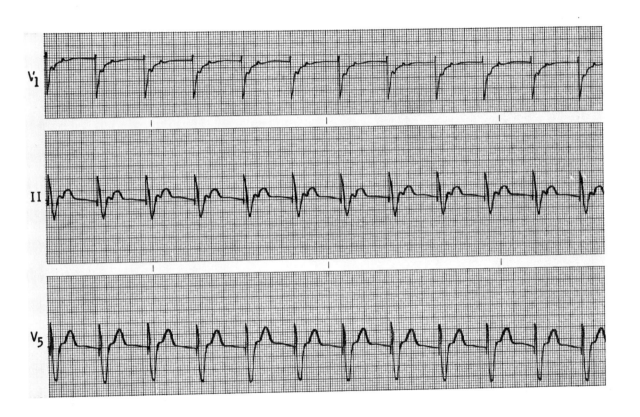

CASE 185: DIAGNOSIS

The cardiac rhythm discloses an artificial pacemaker-induced ventricular rhythm (rate 74 beats per minute) with consecutively occurring atrial capture. That is, the atria are activated in a retrograde fashion.

It should be remembered that this patient received a permanent artificial pacemaker for complete A-V block, but a retrograde conduction may be entirely intact in the presence of complete antegrade (forward) A-V block. This ECG finding is an unequivocal example of unidirectional block.

Needless to say, atrial capture is insignificant clinically in patients with artificial pacemakers.

CASE 186

These cardiac rhythm strips were obtained from a 72-year-old man with a permanent artificial pacemaker.

What is your cardiac rhythm diagnosis?

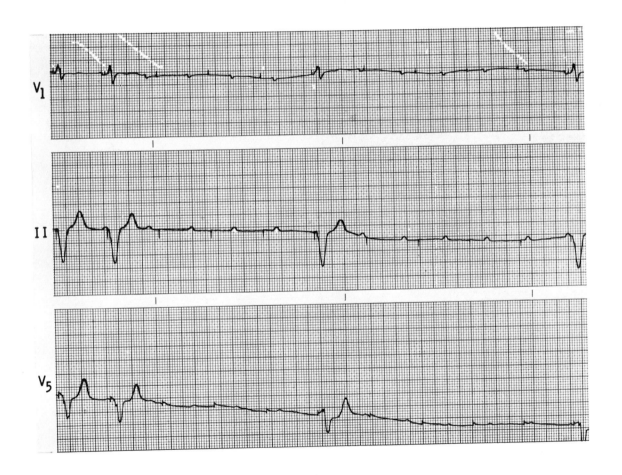

CASE 186: DIAGNOSIS

The basic atrial mechanism is sinus with a rate of 90 beats per minute. Malfunctioning artificial pacemaker is manifested by frequent occurrence of failure of the ventricular capture. Long periods of ventricular standstill are produced because of the failure of the ventricular capture.

The failure of the ventricular capture is most commonly due to malposition of the pacemaker electrode. Less commonly, it may be found in patients with advanced heart disease, fibrosis around the pacemaker electrode, and hyperkalemia. It has been shown that failure of the ventricular capture occasionally occurs during quinidine or procainamide toxicity.

CASE 187

These cardiac rhythm strips were obtained from a 69-year-old man who had had a permanent artificial pacemaker implanted 14 months previously. He was brought to the hospital because of fast pulse rates. Leads II-a, b, and c are not continuous.

1. What is your cardiac rhythm diagnosis?
2. What is the treatment of choice?

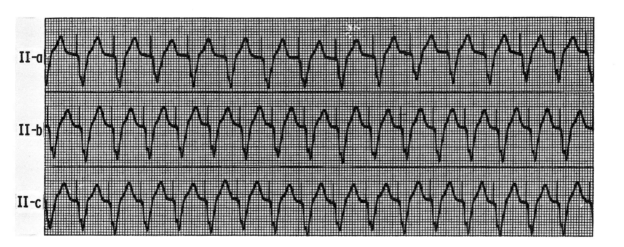

CASE 187: DIAGNOSIS

The atrial mechanism is most likely sinus, but most P waves are not clearly evident. There is an artificial pacemaker-induced ventricular rhythm with a rate of 108–125 beats per minute. It is obvious that the pacing rate is not only faster than the pre-set rate (60 beats per minute), but also the pacing is irregular. This finding is a good example of malfunctioning artificial pacemaker. The malfunction of the pacemaker may be manifested by slowing (see Cases 189 and 190) or acceleration of the pre-set pacing rate (see also Case 188). The acceleration of the pacing rate is termed "runaway pacemaker" which is almost always found in a malfunctioning fixed-rate ventricular pacemaker. Either a slowing or acceleration of the pacing rate may be associated with irregular pacing and/or failure of the ventricular capture (see Cases 186 and 190).

The treatment of choice is immediate discontinuation of the malfunctioning unit. This can be done by cutting the electrode wires near their attachments to the pacemaker. Connecting a temporary pacemaker to the bare electrode ends usually results in prompt recovery of most patients. A new well-functioning permanent unit should be implanted as soon as possible. The runaway pacemaker, needless to say, fails to respond to any antiarrhythmic agent.

CASE 188

A 78-year-old woman who had received a permanent artificial pacemaker implantation 18 months previously for Adams-Stokes syndrome was admitted to the Intermediate Coronary Care Unit because of a fast and irregular heart action.

1. *What is your cardiac rhythm diagnosis?*
2. *What is the treatment of choice?*

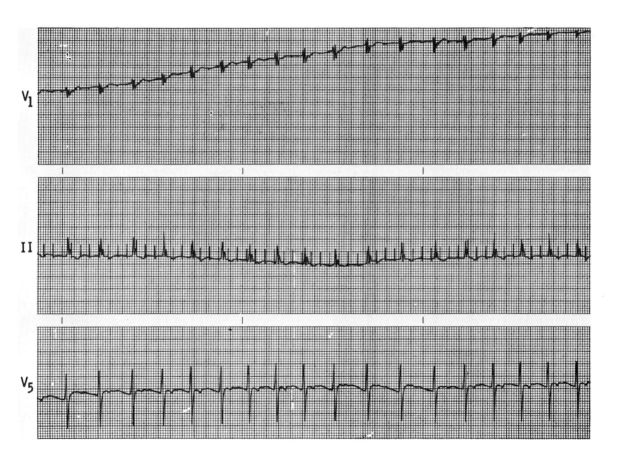

CASE 188: DIAGNOSIS

The underlying cardiac rhythm is atrial fibrillation with rapid ventricular response (ventricular rate 110–130 beats per minute). In addition, there are extremely fast, regularly occurring artificial pacemaker spikes (rate 400 beats per minute) which fail to capture the ventricles. This finding is a typical example of a far-advanced runaway pacemaker—malfunctioning artificial pacemaker (see also Case 187).

As far as the therapeutic approach is concerned, rapid digitalization is the treatment of choice in addition to the replacement of the malfunctioning pacemaker with a new pacemaker as described previously (see Case 187). It must be remembered that any patient may develop various tachyarrhythmias even after the implantation of an artificial pacemaker. Under this circumstance, digitalis and/or other appropriate antiarrhythmic agents may be necessary. In other words, the individual with an artificial pacemaker is by no means immune to the development of any ectopic tachyarrhythmias.

CASE 189

A 74-year-old man was brought to the emergency room because of Adams-Stokes syndrome in spite of a permanent artificial pacemaker which had been implanted 24 months previously.

What is your cardiac rhythm diagnosis?

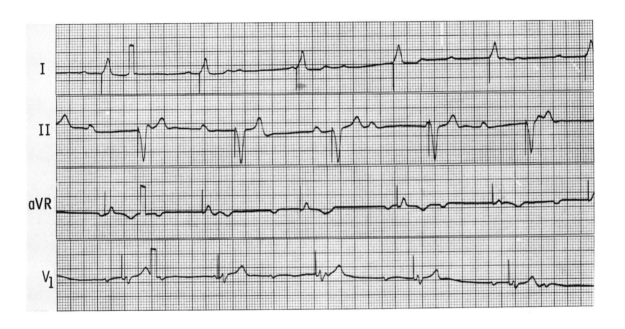

CASE 189: DIAGNOSIS

The cardiac rhythm is sinus (atrial rate 64 beats per minute) with artificial pacemaker-induced ventricular rhythm (ventricular rate 40 beats per minute). Markedly slow pacing rate is obviously a far-advanced malfunctioning pacemaker. The pre-set pacing rate was 70 beats per minute.

CASE 190

These cardiac rhythm strips were obtained from a 70-year-old man with an artificial pacemaker. Malfunction of the artificial pacemaker was suspected.

What is your cardiac rhythm diagnosis?

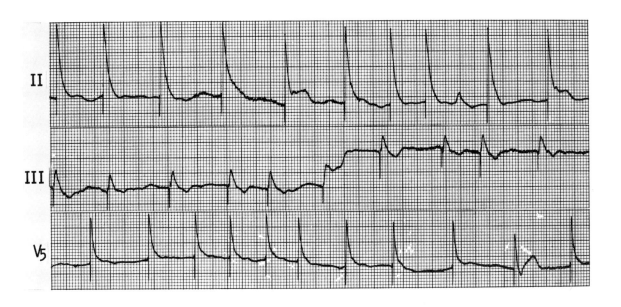

CASE 190: DIAGNOSIS

The atrial mechanism is atrial fibrillation. The malfunctioning pacemaker in this case is manifested by a grossly irregular pacing with rate ranging from 70–130 beats per minute. In general, grossly irregular pacing usually indicates a far-advanced malfunction of the artificial pacemaker.

Various manifestations of malfunction of the artificial pacemakers have been described in detail elsewhere (see Cases 186–189).

CASE 191

These cardiac rhythm strips were obtained from a 79-year-old man who had received a permanent artificial pacemaker 7 months previously.

What is your cardiac rhythm diagnosis?

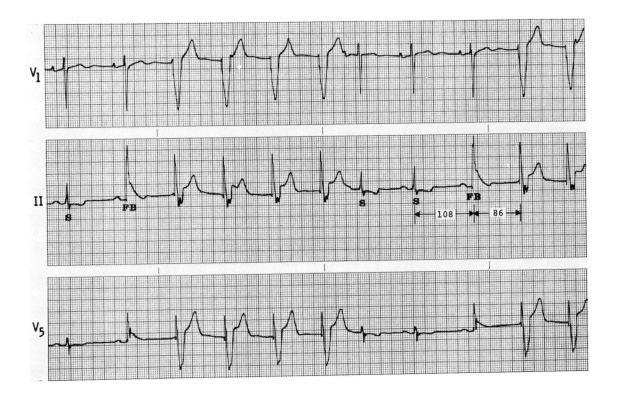

CASE 191: DIAGNOSIS

The tracing shows a ventricular demand pacemaker (Medtronic Model 5943)-induced ventricular rhythm (rate 67 beats per minute) with intermittent sinus beats (marked *S*). Note that the pacemaker escape interval (1.08 seconds) is much longer than the consecutively occurring pacing intervals (0.86 second) because of *hysteresis*. There are occasional ventricular fusion beats (marked *FB*). (The numbers in this figure represent hundredths of a second.)

Hysteresis is a term which describes the difference between the rate at which a pacemaker initiates the pacing and the rate at which it discharges on a consecutive basis. The automatic interval is the time between two successive pacing spikes. The pacemaker escape interval is the length of the period from an intrinsic beat in the patient (sinus or ectopic) to the initial pacing impulse. An example of 10-beat hysteresis would be when a pacemaker does not fire until the patient's rate drops to 60 beats per minute or lower, at which time it starts pacing automatically at 70 beats per minute. This type of hysteresis is seen in the Medtronic Models 5943 and 5843 and the General Electric series A2075.

The only apparent advantage to hysteresis appears in its ability to preserve sinus rhythm. This is accomplished because the patient's own intrinsic rhythm can fall to lower levels (due to the longer escape interval) before asynchronous pacing is initiated. Thus, during rest or sleep when the intrinsic rate tends to be slow, the pacemaker with hysteresis would not fire asynchronously until the rate is reduced below 60 beats per minute. This factor is important only when the patient is in normal sinus rhythm which can occur intermittently in patients with A-V block or other forms of bradyarrhythmias.

There are several disadvantages to hysteresis which should be emphasized. That is, many physicians may misinterpret the hysteresis as a malfunctioning pacemaker because of the difference between the consecutive pacing intervals and the pacemaker escape interval.

Another disadvantage is related to the longer escape interval. After a sensed premature contraction, there is the production of a longer-than-usual postectopic pause which often leads to a longer ineffective ventricular cycle. This is especially true following a ventricular premature contraction.

The effect of hysteresis on battery life of the pacemaker is not yet clear. Although hysteresis does not appear to increase battery drain, the question of whether it increases battery life is unanswered. Part of the problem is due to the fact that the feature of hysteresis may be needed frequently by some patients, and others may never obtain benefit from it.

chapter **13**

MISCELLANEOUS

CASE 192

Renal transplantation was performed for an 18-year-old man with intractable renal failure due to glomerulonephritis.

What is your ECG diagnosis?

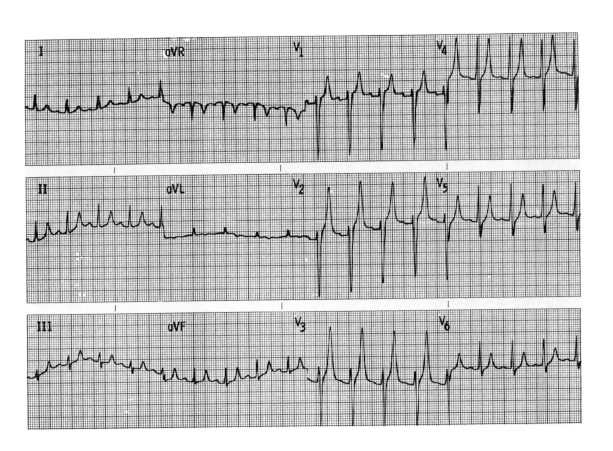

CASE 192: DIAGNOSIS

Cardiac rhythm is sinus tachycardia with a rate of 105 beats per minute.

The striking ECG abnormality in this tracing is a tent-shaped and tall T wave with narrow basis. This T wave change is a typical example of mild to moderately advanced hyperkalemia. His serum potassium level was 7.2 mEq/liter.

It has been well documented that the earliest and the most common ECG abnormality is a tent-shaped and tall T wave practically in all leads, particularly pronounced in leads V_2 through V_4. The T wave change in mild to moderately advanced hyperkalemia (serum potassium 6.0–7.5 mEq/liter) as seen in this case, reveals a narrow base which is a unique feature, distinguished from other ECG abnormalities such as myocardial ischemia, myocarditis, pericarditis, etc. (see Chapters 3 and 4).

When hyperkalemia is further advanced (serum potassium 7.5–8.5 mEq/liter) the P wave amplitude is progressively reduced, and the P wave change is followed by a progressive widening of the QRS complexes leading to eventual absence of the P waves and various intraventricular blocks (see Case 193). In advanced hyperkalemia, varying degree A-V block is often observed. In a far-advanced hyperkalemia (serum potassium 8.5–10 mEq/liter or above), the patient will develop extremely broad QRS complexes with no discernible P waves followed by ventricular tachyarrhythmias, particularly ventricular fibrillation leading to ventricular standstill and even death.

Left ventricular hypertrophy is suggested on this tracing from the voltage criteria (see Case 10).

CASE 193

This electrocardiogram was obtained from a 30-year-old man with far-advanced renal failure. He expired several hours after this ECG tracing was recorded.

What is your ECG diagnosis?

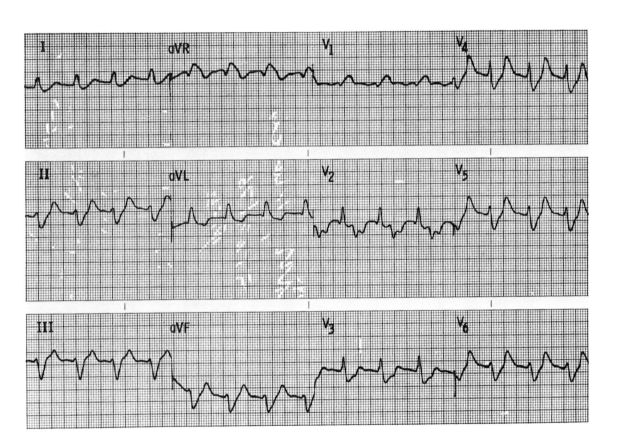

CASE 193: DIAGNOSIS

The cardiac rhythm is sinus rhythm with a rate of 98 beats per minute.

Various manifestations of advanced hyperkalemia are shown in this ECG tracing. They include flat P waves, a bifascicular block consisting of right bundle branch block and left anterior hemiblock (QRS axis −70°), and peaking T waves. The QRS interval is extremely broad in this tracing, and this finding represents diffuse intraventricular block in addition to the bifascicular block (see Chapter 10). In fact, hyperkalemia is one of the most common causes of diffuse (nonspecific) intraventricular block. Bundle branch block, hemiblock, or bifascicular block are much less common than diffuse intraventricular block in advanced hyperkalemia. In addition to various intraventricular blocks, diffuse S-T segment elevation or depression often occurs in advanced hyperkalemia. This hyperkalemia-induced S-T segment alteration may closely resemble an early phase of acute myocardial infarction or acute pericarditis (see Chapters 3 and 4).

His serum potassium was 9.0 mEq/liter when this ECG tracing was taken. His clinical picture further deteriorated rapidly, and he finally developed ventricular fibrillation followed by ventricular standstill which was irreversible.

Various ECG abnormalities in hyperkalemia have been described elsewhere (see Case 92).

CASE 194

A 66-year-old man was admitted to the hospital because of severe diarrhea.

What is your ECG diagnosis?

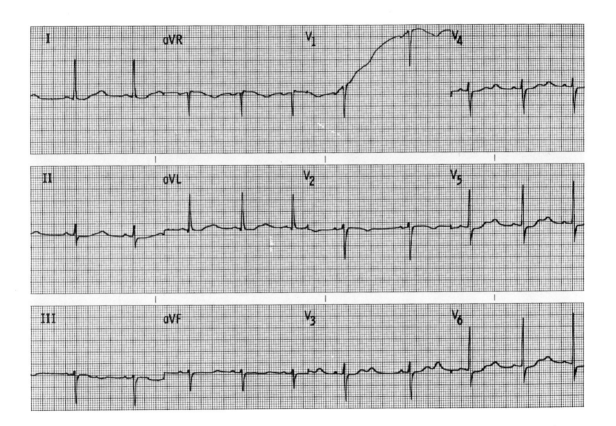

CASE 194: DIAGNOSIS

The cardiac rhythm is sinus arrhythmia and areas of sinus bradycardia with rate ranging from 55–68 beats per minute.

It is readily recognized that the amplitude of the U wave is markedly increased. When the amplitude of the U wave is equal to or exceeds the T wave amplitude, the term "prominent U wave" is used. The prominent U wave is most pronounced in leads V_2 through V_5 in most cases. The prominent U wave is considered to be almost a pathognomonic feature of hypokalemia. His serum potassium level was 3.0 mEq/liter.

It can be said that the prominent U wave is the earliest and most common ECG abnormality in mild hypokalemia. When the potassium level is further reduced (serum potassium below 3.0 mEq/liter), the prominent U wave is followed by a peaking P wave (pseudo-P-pulmonale). In severe hypokalemia, the patient may develop various cardiac arrhythmias, and it may even cause death.

It has been repeatedly emphasized that hypokalemia frequently predisposes to digitalis intoxication.

The prominent U wave often coexists with a low amplitude of the T wave, and even flat or inverted T wave may be observed in hypokalemia. The prominent U wave due to hypokalemia may resemble a prolonged Q-T interval when the U wave is misinterpreted as a broad T wave (a sum of the T wave and the U wave).

CASE 195

This ECG tracing was obtained from a 17-year-old girl with Ewing's sarcoma.

What is your ECG diagnosis?

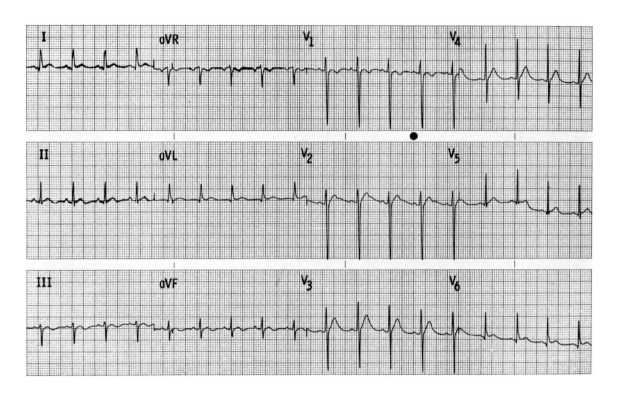

CASE 195: DIAGNOSIS

The cardiac rhythm is sinus tachycardia with a rate of 110 beats per minute.

The striking ECG abnormality in this tracing is a short Q-T interval due to a virtual absence of the S-T segment. This ECG finding is a unique feature of hypercalcemia.

It should be noted that digitalis and calcium have a synergistic action. Therefore, digitalization should be carried out with extreme care when digitalis is considered to be absolutely indicated in the presence of hypercalcemia. The smallest dosage of digitalis should be tried under this circumstance in order to avoid digitalis toxicity. Sudden death has been reported following digitalization in the patient with hypercalcemia. Thus, digitalis should be avoided whenever possible in the presence of hypercalcemia.

CASE 196

A 24-year-old woman was admitted to the Renal Service for a periodic hemodialysis for chronic renal failure.

What is your ECG diagnosis?

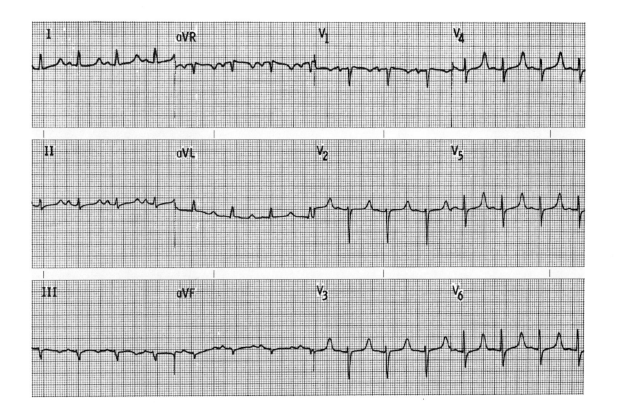

CASE 196: DIAGNOSIS

The cardiac rhythm is sinus with a rate of 90 beats per minute.

There are two coexisting ECG abnormalities due to hyperkalemia and hypocalcemia. Hyperkalemia and hypocalcemia often coexist in a patient with advanced renal failure.

The ECG abnormality due to hyperkalemia is obviously peaked T waves which are pronounced in leads V_2 through V_6 (see Case 192).

The hypocalcemia-induced ECG change is a markedly prolonged Q-T interval as a result of a lengthening of the S-T segment. Thus, the lengthening of the S-T segment is a unique and primary feature of hypocalcemia, and the prolonged Q-T interval is the end result of the S-T segment alteration.

CASE 197

A 36-year-old obese woman who has been taking birth control pills for several years was seen in the emergency room because of severe chest pain associated with marked dyspnea. She had been perfectly healthy prior to this episode.

What is your ECG diagnosis?

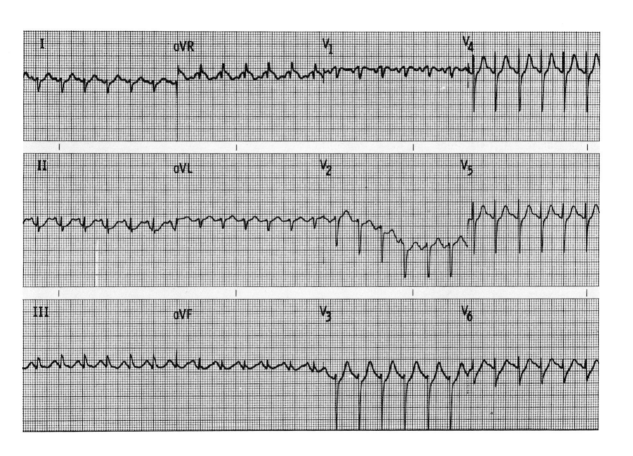

CASE 197: DIAGNOSIS

The cardiac rhythm is marked sinus tachycardia with a rate of 156 beats per minute.

This tracing reveals various ECG abnormalities which include right axis deviation of the QRS complexes (QRS axis +120°), posterior axis deviation of the QRS complexes, P-pulmonale, and a pseudo-diaphragmatic myocardial infarction pattern. These ECG changes are typical features of acute pulmonary embolism. Among these ECG abnormalities, sinus tachycardia and right axis deviation are probably the earliest and the most common findings in pulmonary embolism. In addition, there is a low voltage of the QRS complexes (see Case 32).

Various manifestations of pulmonary embolism are summarized as follows:

1. Marked sinus tachycardia (most common).
2. Right axis deviation of the QRS complexes (most common).
3. P-pulmonale (common).
4. Inverted T waves in leads V_1 through V_3 (relatively common).
5. Pseudo-diaphragmatic myocardial ischemia or infarction pattern (relatively common).
6. Posterior axis deviation of the QRS complexes (relatively common).
7. S_1, Q_3 pattern (less common).
8. Right bundle branch block of acute onset—often transient (less common).
9. Transient atrial tachyarrhythmias (less common).
10. Diffuse S-T, T wave changes (less common).

It has been well documented that the thromboembolic phenomenon, particularly pulmonary embolism, is relatively common in women who are taking birth control pills.

CASE 198

This electrocardiogram was obtained from a 26-year-old man who was referred to a cardiologist for the diagnosis of his heart disease. Echocardiogram confirmed the clinical as well as the electrocardiographic diagnosis on this patient.

1. What is your ECG diagnosis?
2. What is the underlying heart disease?

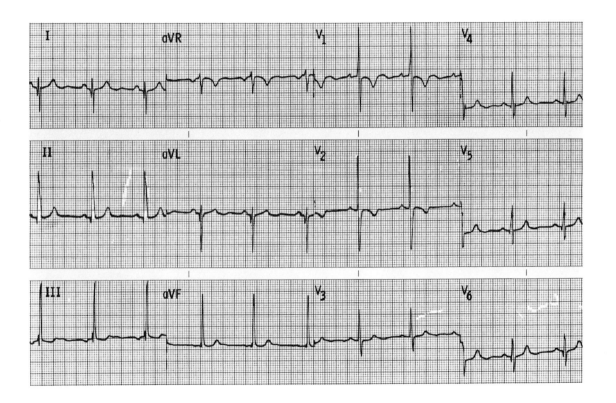

CASE 198: DIAGNOSIS

The cardiac rhythm is sinus with a rate of 64 beats per minute.

The striking ECG abnormalities in this tracing include tall R waves in leads V_1 and V_2 and narrow Q waves in leads I, aVL, and V_5 and V_6, with marked reduction of the R wave amplitude in these left precordial leads. These ECG findings closely mimic posterolateral myocardial infarction including high lateral wall involvement. However, this pseudo-myocardial infarction pattern is considered to be due to a ventricular septal hypertrophy in idiopathic hypertrophic subaortic stenosis (IHSS). The diagnosis of IHSS was confirmed by echocardiogram on this patient.

Note inverted T waves in leads V_1 and V_2 which represent the juvenile T wave pattern (see Case 2).

It has been well documented that IHSS is one of the most common causes of a pseudo-myocardial infarction pattern.

CASE 199

Two ECG tracings shown on this page (tracing A) and on the next page (tracing B) were obtained from a 71-year-old man with no apparent heart disease.

What is your ECG diagnosis?

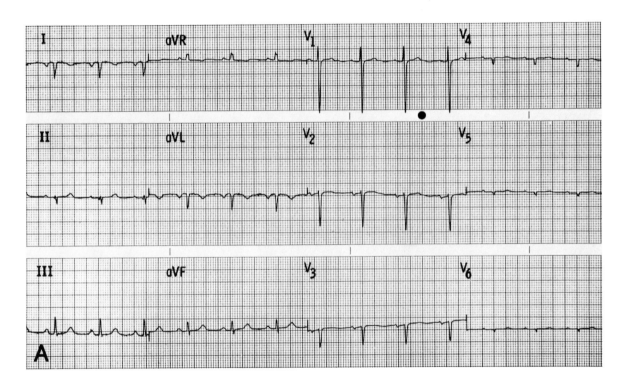

CASE 199: DIAGNOSIS

The ECG tracing A appears to be taken with reversed electrodes between the left and right arms, because the entire P, QRS, and T complexes are inverted in lead I, and leads aVR and aVL appear to be switched. However, by close observation, the precordial leads also look grossly abnormal. That is, the R wave amplitude is progressively reduced from lead V_1 toward the left precordium with eventual loss of the R waves (Q-S pattern) and very small QRS complexes in leads V_4 through V_6. These ECG findings are typical features seen in patients with a mirror-image dextrocardia.

It should be noted that the morphology of the entire P–QRS–T complexes shown in the right precordial leads (leads V_{2R} through V_{6R}) is completely within normal limits (tracing B).

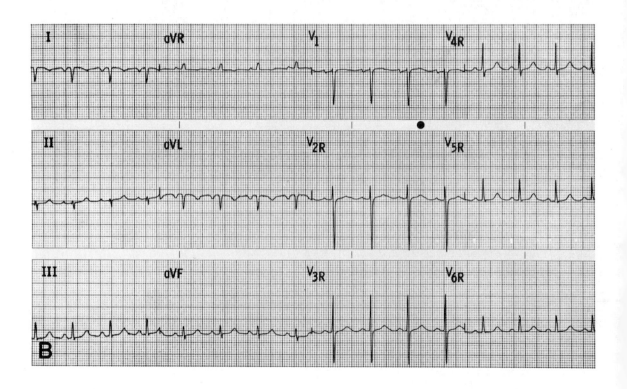

CASE 200

The ECG tracing was obtained from a 70-year-old man with coronary heart disease.

What is your cardiac rhythm diagnosis?

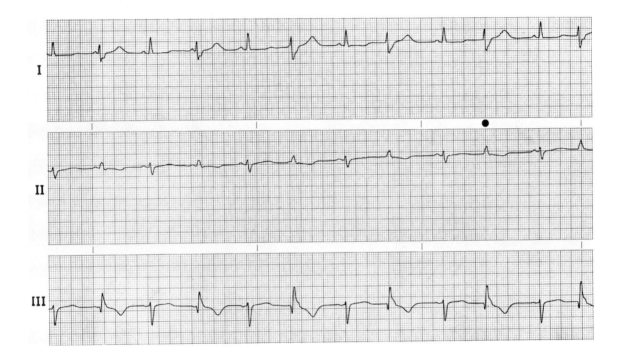

CASE 200: DIAGNOSIS

The underlying cardiac rhythm is sinus with a rate of 67 beats per minute.

There are frequent ventricular ectopic beats which occur alternately with the basic beats causing ventricular bigeminy. This ECG finding superficially appears to be frequent ventricular premature contractions.

However, by close observation, the diagnosis of ventricular parasystole can be entertained on the basis of varying coupling intervals, constant shortest interectopic intervals with frequent ventricular fusion beats (the first and second ventricular ectopic beats). The rate of the ventricular parasystole is 34 beats per minute. Detailed descriptions regarding parasystole are found elsewhere (see Case 85).

In addition, there is the evidence of left anterior hemiblock (QRS axis −45°, calculated from a 12-lead ECG; see Chapter 10).

Suggested Reading

Chung EK: Digitalis Intoxication. Amsterdam, Excerpta Medica, 1969

Chung EK: Electrocardiography: Practical Applications with Vectorial Principles, Hagerstown, Harper & Row, 1974

Chung EK: Vectorcardiography: Self Assessment. Hagerstown, Harper & Row, 1974

Chung EK: Clinical Electrocardiography (Part 5), Cardiac Arrhythmias: Differential Diagnosis. New York, Medcom, 1975

Chung EK: Wolff–Parkinson–White syndrome: Current views. Am J Med 62:252, 1977

Chung EK: Principles of Cardiac Arrhythmias, 2nd ed. Baltimore, William & Wilkins, 1977

Chung EK, Chung LS: Carotid Sinus Stimulation in Non-Invasive Cardiac Diagnosis. Philadelphia, Lea & Febiger, 1976

Cohen HC, Rosen KM, Pick A: Disorders of impulse conduction and impulse formation caused by hyperkalemia in man. Am Heart J 89:501, 1975

Ferrer MI: Pre-Excitation. New York, Futura, 1976

Furman S, Escher DJW: Modern Cardiac Pacing. A Clinical Overview. Bowie, Charles Press, 1975

Krikler DM, Goodwin JF: Cardiac Arrhythmias. The Modern Electrophysiological Approach. Philadelphia, WB Saunders, 1975

Marcus FI: Current concepts of digoxin therapy. Mod. Concepts Cardiovas Dis 45:77, 1976

Marriott HJL: Practical Electrocardiography, 6th ed. Baltimore, Williams & Wilkins, 1977

Narula OS: His Bundle Electrocardiography and Clinical Electrophysiology. Philadelphia, FA Davis, 1975

O'Neil JP, Chung EK: Unusual electrocardiographic findings: bifascicular block due to hyperkalemia. Am J Med 61:537, 1976

Resnekov L: Symposium on Cardiac Rhythm Disturbances. I. The Medical Clinics of North America, Vol 60. Philadelphia, WB Saunders, 1976

Resnekov L: Symposium on Cardiac Rhythm Disturbances. II. The Medical Clinics of North America, Vol 60. Philadelphia, WB Saunders, 1976

Surawicz B: Electrolytes and the electrocardiogram. Mod Concept Cardiovas Dis 33:875, 1964

Wellens HJJ, Lie KI, Janse MJ: The Conduction System of The Heart. Philadelphia, Lea & Febiger, 1976

Index

Numbers refer to case presentations

Aberrant ventricular conduction, 76, 79, 84, 85, 87, 88, 95, 124

Adams-Stokes syndrome, 144, 165, 167

Angina pectoris. *See* Myocardial ischemia, injury, and infarction
 Prinzmetal's angina, 33

Aortocoronary bypass surgery. *See* Post-cardiotomy syndrome

Arrhythmias related to artificial pacemakers, 129, 177–191
 artificial pacemaker. *See* Arrhythmias related to artificial pacemakers
 artificial pacemaker escape-bigeminy, 180
 artificial pacemaker malfunction, 81, 186–190
 atrial pacemaker rhythm, 181
 atrial-synchronized pacemaker rhythm, 183
 bifocal demand pacemaker rhythm, 184
 coronary sinus pacemaker rhythm, 182
 demand (ventricular) pacemaker rhythm, 178–180, 191
 fixed-rate (ventricular) pacemaker rhythm, 177
 pacemaker hysteresis, 178, 191
 pacemaker rhythm with atrial capture, 185

Ashman's phenomenon, 88. *See also* Aberrant ventricular conduction

Atrial arrhythmias, 83–111
 atrial fibrillation, 12, 13, 17, 22, 23, 40, 70, 107–110, 119, 122, 125, 127, 138, 152, 176, 188, 190
 atrial flutter-fibrillation, 117
 atrial flutter, 20, 96–106, 142, 175
 atrial premature contractions, 21, 83–90, 96
  atrial bigeminy, 83, 87, 88
  blocked (nonconducted), 85, 86
  with aberrant ventricular conduction, 84, 85, 87, 88
 atrial tachycardia, 89, 90, 92–95, 111, 118, 178
  multifocal, 94–95
  with A-V block, 92–93
  with A-V junctional tachycardia, 111, 118

Atrial hypertrophy (enlargement). *See* Chamber enlargement
 left atrial hypertrophy, 11, 12, 16, 17, 25, 110, 165
 right atrial hypertrophy, 18, 19, 21

Atrial septal defect, 27, 61, 63, 141
 ostium primum type, 141
 ostium secundum type, 27, 61, 63

Atrioventricular (A-V) conduction disturbances: 130–144
 advanced A-V block, 125, 138, 149, 167, 178
 A-V block. *See* A-V conduction disturbances
 complete (third degree) A-V block, 20, 105, 127, 139, 144
 first degree A-V block, 11, 57, 130, 165
 high degree A-V block. *See* Advanced A-V block
 Mobitz type I A-V block. *See* Wenckebach A-V block
 Mobitz type II A-V block, 136, 167, 179
 3:1 A-V block, 137
 2:1 A-V block, 93, 134, 135, 180
 Wenckebach A-V block, 92, 123, 124, 131–133, 137

Atrioventricular (A-V) junctional arrhythmias: 112–129
 A-V dissociation, 23, 76, 111, 116–120, 122, 129, 139, 141–144, 150, 152
 A-V junctional escape beats and rhythm, 20, 125–128, 139–143, 149
 A-V junctional escape bigeminy, 77
 A-V junctional premature contractions, 112
  A-V junctional bigeminy, 112
 A-V junctional tachycardia
  non-paroxysmal, 23, 111, 115–122, 129
  paroxysmal, 113, 114, 123

A-V nodal. *See* A-V junctional

Barlow's syndrome. *See* Mitral valve prolapse syndrome

Bidirectional ventricular tachycardia, 150, 152

Bifascicular block, 77, 141, 163, 164, 166, 193

Bifocal demand pacemaker rhythm, 184

Bilateral bundle branch block. *See* Bifascicular block, trifascicular block, and complete A-V block

Biventricular hypertrophy, 22, 23, 24

Cardiomyopathy, 67, 68, 72, 97, 104, 151
Carditis. *See* Myocarditis and pericarditis
Carotid sinus stimulation, 78, 91
  hypersensitive carotid sinus syndrome, 78
Chamber enlargement (hypertrophy), 10–27
Chest deformity, 19
Chronic obstructive pulmonary disease. *See* Cor-pulmonale
Coarse atrial fibrillation, 12, 17, 22, 110, 138
Congenital heart disease, 15, 20, 24, 27, 31, 61, 63, 64, 74, 105, 141
Coronary heart disease. *See* Myocardial ischemia, injury and infarction
Coronary insufficiency, 28
Coronary sinus pacemaker rhythm, 182
Cor-pulmonale, 18, 19, 21, 94, 95, 98, 99

Dextrocardia, 199
Digitalis effect, 106, 115
Digitalis intoxication, 23, 76, 77, 92, 116, 117, 118, 119, 122, 125, 127, 129, 130, 131, 138, 142, 143, 146, 149, 152
Disturbances of sinus impulse formation and conduction, 71–82
Dressler's syndrome, 60

Early repolarization pattern, 3
Electrical alternans, 113
Electrolyte imbalances, 13, 16, 40, 192–196
Escape-bigeminy, 77, 137, 180
Exercise ECG test, 30
  false positive test, 31
  positive test, 30
Exit block, 122
Ewing's sarcoma, 195

First degree A-V block. *See* A-V block
Fixed-rate artificial pacemaker, 177

Giant T wave syndrome, 28

Hemiblocks. *See* Left anterior and posterior hemiblock
High degree A-V block. *See* A-V block
Holter monitor electrocardiogram, 90, 173
Hypercalcemia, 195
Hyperkalemia, 192, 193, 196
Hypocalcemia, 196
Hypokalemia, 13, 16, 40, 194
Hysteresis, 178, 191

Idiopathic hypertrophic subaortic stenosis (IHSS), 198
Intermittent left bundle branch block, 161
Intermittent right bundle branch block, 159
Intermittent Wolff-Parkinson-White syndrome, 172
Intraventricular conduction disturbances, 155–167
  bifascicular block, 77, 141, 163, 164, 166, 193
  diffuse, 52, 72, 193
  hemiblocks, 29, 40, 41, 96, 99, 136, 155, 156, 157, 163, 164, 165, 166, 193
  left bundle branch block, 108, 146, 160
  right bundle branch block, 26, 59, 109, 114, 158, 162, 163, 164, 165, 166, 175, 193
  trifascicular block, 136, 144, 165, 167

Junctional. *See* A-V junctional
Juvenile T wave pattern, 2, 4, 5, 6, 24, 57

Left anterior hemiblock, 29, 40, 41, 96, 99, 119, 126, 155, 156
Left atrial hypertrophy, 11, 12, 16, 17, 25, 110, 165
Left axis deviation of P waves, 8
Left bundle branch block, 108, 146
Left posterior hemiblock, 157
Left ventricular hypertrophy, 10, 11, 13, 25, 26, 34, 40, 44, 49, 50, 93, 100, 103, 117, 127, 130
  diastolic overloading pattern, 14
  systolic overloading pattern. *See* Left ventricular hypertrophy

Low voltage, 32, 37, 38, 39, 43, 69, 70, 113, 162
Lupus erythematosus induced by Pronestyl, 59

Mitral stenosis, 12, 16, 17, 22, 110
Mitral valve prolapse syndrome, 31
Myocardial Injury, 32
   subendocardial injury, 32
   subepicardial injury, 33
Myocardial ischemia, injury and infarction, 28–53
   anterior, 41
   anteroseptal, 35, 36, 37, 51, 111, 118, 162, 164, 166
   diaphragmatic, 25, 38, 42, 43, 46, 49, 50, 51, 52, 60, 66,
      111, 120, 123, 133, 134, 137, 139, 140, 162
   diaphragmatic-lateral, 44, 132, 135, 181
   diaphragmatic-postero-lateral, 48, 65
   extensive anterior, 38, 39, 40, 52, 53, 156, 179
   high lateral, 41, 47
   posterior, 45, 46, 50, 100
   postero-lateral, 47, 136
   pseudo myocardial infarction pattern, 19, 168, 170, 173,
      176, 198
Myocardial ischemia, 28, 29, 30, 34, 92
   diffuse, 28, 29, 51, 92, 148, 155, 159
   posterior, 30, 43
Myocarditis and pericarditis, 54–70
   rheumatic, 57
   viral, 58

Nodal arrhythmias. *See* A-V junctional arrhythmias
Nodal escape rhythm. *See* A-V junctional escape rhythm
Nodal premature contraction. *See* A-V junctional prema-
   ture contraction
Nodal tachycardia. *See* A-V junctional tachycardia
Nonspecific S-T, T wave change, 21, 94
Normal electrocardiogram, 1, 71, 73, 75
Normal sinus rhythm, 1, 7, 9, 10, 11, 14, 16, 18, 25, 27,
   28, 33, 35, 36, 39, 41, 43, 45, 48, 51, 52, 59, 60, 62,
   63, 66, 156, 157, 160, 163, 164, 168
Normal variants, 1–9

Pacemaker. *See* Artificial Pacemaker
Parasystole, 85, 151, 200

PAT. *See* Atrial tachycardia
PAT with block. *See* Atrial tachycardia with A-V block
Patent ductus arteriosus, 24
Pericarditis, 54–70
   bacterial, 56
   idiopathic, 54
   pericardial effusion, 69, 70, 113
   pronestyl-induced, 59
   rheumatoid, 70
   traumatic, 56
   viral, 55
Post-cardiotomy syndrome, 61, 62, 63, 64, 65, 66
Post-ectopic T wave change, 148
Post-myocardial infarction syndrome. *See* Dressler's syn-
   drome
Post-operative arrhythmias, 105, 115, 121, 141
Post-operative A-V block, 105, 141
P-pulmonale, 18, 19, 21
Prinzmetal's angina, 33
Pseudo myocardial infarction pattern, 19, 168, 170, 173,
   176, 198
Pseudo ventricular tachycardia, 176
Pulmonary embolism, 197
Pulmonic stenosis, 15, 64, 74

Quinidine effect, 103, 104, 115

Reciprocating tachycardia, 123, 124
   in Wolff-Parkinson-White syndrome, 174
Renal failure, 192, 193, 196
Retrograde ventriculoatrial block, 126
Rheumatic fever, 57
Right atrial hypertrophy, 18, 19, 21
Right axis deviation, 9, 12, 15, 16, 17, 19, 20, 22, 27, 63,
   64, 197
Right bundle branch block, 26, 59, 109, 114, 135, 136, 158,
   159, 162, 175
   associated with hemiblocks. *See* Bifascicular block
   intermittent, 159
   right bundle branch block pattern, 27, 61

Right ventricular hypertrophy, 12, 15, 16, 17, 18, 19, 20, 27, 63, 74, 98, 105, 110
R-on-T phenomenon, 29, 154, 177
Runaway pacemaker, 81, 187, 188

Sarcoidosis, 67
Second degree A-V block. *See* A-V block
Short P-R interval, 7, 42, 65
Sickle cell anemia, 68
Sick sinus syndrome, 79, 80
Sinoatrial (S-A) block
  Mobitz type I (Wenckebach), 82
  Mobitz type II, 80, 81
Sinus arrest, 78, 79
Sinus Arrhythmias. *See* Disturbances of sinus impulse formation and conduction
Sinus arrhythmia, 2, 5, 15, 42, 57, 73, 74, 170, 173
Sinus bradycardia, 3, 6, 24, 26, 34, 50, 75, 76, 77, 120, 159, 173
Sinus tachycardia, 4, 19, 21, 24, 37, 38, 49, 55, 56, 58, 61, 64, 67, 69, 71, 72, 96, 197
Supraventricular tachycardia, 91

Transposition of the great vessels, 20, 105
Trifascicular block, 136, 144, 165, 167

U wave. *See* Hypokalemia
  inverted U wave, 34

Ventricular aneurysm, 53
Ventricular arrhythmias, 145–154
  during exercise, 30
  interpolated, 148
  post-ectopic T wave change, 148
  R-on-T phenomenon, 29, 154
  ventricular bigeminy, 30, 125, 145, 146, 149
  ventricular escape beats, 137, 138, 149
  ventricular escape bigeminy, 137
  ventricular escape rhythm, 144, 167
  ventricular fibrillation, 154, 176
  ventricular flutter, 153
  ventricular parasystole, 200
  ventricular premature contractions, 29, 30, 90, 122, 145, 146, 147, 148, 149, 154, 181, 182
  ventricular quadrigeminy, 29, 148
  ventricular tachycardia, 150, 151, 152
    bidirectional, 150, 152
    parasystolic, 151
Ventricular trigeminy, 147
Ventricular pre-excitation syndrome. *See* WPW syndrome

Wandering atrial pacemaker, 74
Wenckebach A-V block. *See* A-V block
Wenckebach A-V response in atrial flutter, 101–103, 175
Wenckebach exit block, 122
Wenckebach S-A block. *See* S-A block
Wolff-Parkinson-White (WPW) syndrome, 168–176
  atrial fibrillation, 176
  atrial flutter, 175
  intermittent, 172
  reciprocating tachycardia, 174
  with multiple pathways, 173